Prairie Fire

A Guidebook for
Surviving Civil War 2

Clay Martin

Dedication

For all the unsung heroes of the GWOT, and before.
I fear your skills may
once again be needed.
For a cause not of our choosing.

And for Saint Rittenhouse,
Hero of Kenosha,
Defender of the Realm.
They are going to make a statue of you one day son.
Unfortunately, they might make you a martyr before that.

Cover by @spy_sapper
Editing by Horus Pitchfork
Much appreciated ninjas!

Table of Contents

Introduction

Welcome to Prairie Fire—the spiritual successor to *Concrete Jungle: A Green Beret's Guide to Urban Survival.* Prairie Fire is a term with many meanings. First off, if you have ever lived on the plains, you know just how fast and destructive a prairie fire can be. A forest fire might burn hotter, but nothing on God's green Earth can match the speed of flames in a sea of three foot tall grass whipped on by sixty to seventy mile-per-hour winds. It can be on you and burn you out before 'quit and get ready.' Lightning in the sky always brings watchers to the windows because a single strike can torch everything you own in a heartbeat if you aren't on your game. The second meaning comes from MACV-SOG in the Vietnam War. "Prairie Fire" was a brevity code for the radio that meant a Recon Team was in danger of being overrun. Those two words diverted all available air support in theater to rain bombs from the sky, and spun up a Mike or Hatchet Force to come put the curb stomp on (a Mike or Hatchet Force was a company-sized element of ass kickers lead by Green Berets—a theater level Quick Reaction Force). In Special Forces, we pay tribute to the giants on whose shoulders we stand. Prairie Fire also fits quite well with the predicament rural America finds itself in today.

I struggled with choosing this title and not because it isn't appropriate. I almost backed out of it because it is also the title of the Weather Underground's political manifesto published in the

'70s. Well fuck that—we are taking our words back! Bill Ayers and the rest of his kind can argue about it in Hell. If this year plays out the way I think it might, that reunion will be sooner rather than later.

The proverbial doody hasn't hit the fan yet but it is definitely on trajectory and speed. I have never seen anything like this and I doubt any of you have either. In *Concrete Jungle*, I made a point of saying that we hadn't reached '70s level bombings and assassinations yet—I also had the benefit of writing it in 2019. What we have seen so far is an escalation I would have thought unimaginable. Methinks the Commies learned something from the last go-round and have adapted tactics. As I sit here, Portland has had nightly riots for over seventy days. Multiple attempts have been made to burn down the Federal Courthouse there. Dozens of our major cities have been looted and burned out while the police forces have been ordered to let it happen. District Attorneys nationwide have released the few arrested with no charges. Last night, a man was murdered by a mob in cold blood. In the span of nine months we have gone from, "maybe you should kinda get ready, just in case" to "war is on the horizon; make peace with your god because some of you will meet him shortly. I hope you packed clean socks."

That also changes the information I am putting in this volume. *Concrete Jungle* was written with the idea that you had time to get it together. You had time to get specialized training. You could move your chess pieces into position. You could buy all the guns and training ammo you wanted (if you failed to stock up, that's not a funny joke). The message here is much more urgent. If *Concrete Jungle* was waves lapping ashore, slowly increasing in volume to wake you up, *Prairie Fire* is a dive klaxon on top of a Drill Instructor inches from your face screaming, *"On your feet, shitstick! Drop your cocks and grab your socks!"* or, you know, whatever they say to the chicks on Parris Island (someone send an email, I really do want to know what the female version of that is).

If you have the first volume, you may notice that I have shifted my tone and language. Yeah, guilty as charged. *Concrete Jungle*, while from the heart and written to relay important information, was also envisioned as something that might be commercially viable and apolitical. That ship has sailed. This is about the battle for the soul of our country—the world my children grow up in. Not the cutesy way politicians say "battle for the soul of our country" on the way to sell us out for a couple of bucks and a trip to Epstein Island, I mean the streets are going to run red with blood one way or another and I have a vested fucking interest in making sure my team wins. So forgive my lack of niceties and tact. It is faster for me to type "rip his goddamn lungs out his pee hole" than it is to think of a proper-sounding phrase. I was raised by savages so it's the way I think. It's also the way I would talk if I was standing in front of you delivering a lesson on how not to get killed.

You are also going to find that my advice for rural survival in the upcoming animated contest for liberty is much more logistics based than my urban survival book. There's a simple reason for that. The best thing you can do if a city is plunged into civil war is to leave. Those of us in the rural areas don't have that luxury. If the fight comes to us, there is nowhere else to go. You are the last line of defense on the entire planet for freedom. Europe has already had its nuts cut off by hate speech laws and an endless flow of migrant "youth." Australia is so cucked that it might as well be

France. Canada is busy stripping the last of its rights from the populace via executive order—at least when the Prime Minister isn't busy dressing up in black face or going on sabbaticals to India.

Please read the entire book before you start spending your kids' inheritance. If you start with nothing and try to buy everything I recommend, you could spend the next four months just shopping, which isn't necessary. I am trying to cover all the bases for you so that you can make an educated decision. One thing you absolutely should do is sit down and think about what you actually need. I also want you to keep one specific thing in mind. In fact, highlight the following sentence, mark the page and refer to it often, especially when it's time to get "stuff."

I would rather have a fit man with an obsolete Chinesium rifle he has fired 5,000 rounds through than a weak man equipped with the latest load out for Seal Team 6 that he hasn't trained with!

Now some of you aren't familiar with me so let me go ahead and break some hearts right here: I don't pull punches and you already bought my book, so I have nothing to lose. I am going to tell you some things that you don't want to hear because it takes you out of your comfortable belief bubble. I am going to say some things that may be downright insulting. I'd rather hurt some feelings up front than have you die face down in the sand unnecessarily. If you hear me out, with an open mind, I think you will find that what I am telling you is true. Maybe not 100% across the board, but in general it will be correct.

This is a good place to give you my rural bonafides. I grew up on a dirt road, had a moto-cross track in the backyard and lived in a trailer house that was blown away by a tornado. If that ain't country, it'll hair lip the pope (and if you don't know those lyrics, your right to challenge my résumé just went out the window).

How about my qualifications to teach you tactics? Glad you asked. I am a career military dude, having served in two branches. I was a USMC Infantryman, Recon Marine and Scout Sniper, then I cross decked into US Army Special Forces where I did all kinds of silly shit. I was a sniper in a direct action unit, an assaulter in the same, taught CQB and was also involved in some weirdo intelligence ninja stuff. In fact, I am not just a ruggedly handsome door kicker, I was also an 18F Special Forces Intelligence Sergeant. I have operated all over the world in maybe every clime and place. As a Green Beret, I have turned illiterate peasants and dirt worshiping heathens with a 3rd grade education into functional armies—it's kinda what we do. I can help you. I was also trained to ignore pain and eat things that would make a billy goat puke... (feel free to ignore that, I am contractually obligated to say it once per book. It's out of the way now).

Lets dive in, shall we?

1   Getting Your Poop in One Bag

I spent a lot of time in *Concrete Jungle* talking about organization and team building. I hate to break it to you, but 'one man against the world' just doesn't work. If you try going all Johnny Rambo solo operator in the coming shenanigans, you are just gonna get killed; probably rather quickly. The real world just doesn't work that way. Compared to most humans, my last two decades of experience reads like a demon's résumé and I can't do it alone either—nor will I try.

Even among Team guys, we know that we get exponentially more dangerous the more of us there are. 1+1=3 but also 2+1=7... No, that isn't new Lefty approved math, it means that two of us might equal three mortals, but three of us equal seven and all twelve of us are a force to be reckoned with well out of proportion to our numbers. Some of that is just due to simple solutions to problems. One dude can only do so much but two of you? Now you can do basic Fire and Maneuver with one shooting while the other moves. Three makes for overwatch or a flanking element. Maybe it just means you can eat a sandwich while someone else stands guard; that has a very real value as well.

Concrete Jungle laid out a plan for building your own ODA (Operational Detachment Alpha or A-Team) which is still a structure

I stand by. It is flexible and agile, and a great way to load skill sets. I will put that chapter up on my website (off-the-reservation.com) so that we don't have to fully rehash it here.

To simplify things, I would approach it like this: right now, you want to build and recruit a team of specialists in a four to six man cell. Up to twelve is great if you can field it, but that is unlikely. For most practical applications that just becomes two separate six man teams anyway. We start here because no matter the rhetoric, no matter the initial excitement, you are going have a really hard time gathering more than that who are really down for the cause. If you start out with twenty, half won't show up by the second training session. By the third you'll be hearing about how the "wife won't let me out this weekend" or "I need to stay home and iron the cat." If the random strap hangers do show up later, you'll spend half your time catching them up to speed. It will be an anchor chained to the solid people in the crew and ultimately an exercise in futility.

You need to find a couple of people that are mentally tough, dedicated and most importantly, true believers in what is about to unfold. If you are starting from scratch now, sacrifices of both time and treasure are going to be needed to be ready by go time. This isn't the time for fence-sitters, at least in the inner circle. You may also end up "chalk talking" some eventualities that are not for public consumption. I'm talking far in the future type events if law and order has completely broken down. You need to think about such things, but it's probably best not to have them spread all over Facebook or the wives' sewing circle. You need people with some goddamn sense, which is often in short supply.

I said this in the last book but it bears reiteration: anyone that starts talking about making bombs, illegal SBRs, machine guns or suppressors is a Fed. If they aren't a Fed, they are still going to get you pinched by the Feds. Uncle Sugar does not fuck around with that silliness. Such a person should immediately be cast out of the group and shunned. Frame this and put it on the wall where ever you do your meetings.

Your four to six man team, simply referred to as a team or Team hereafter, is your core formation. These are people you are tight with and can rely on. This is where you want to spend the majority of your training time going forward and where you want to invest your training dollars. As we will discuss in subsequent chapters, you may have to pool funds for some specialized training. If you can only send one person, make sure it is a person worth sending.

While you have a smaller overall talent pool to draw from, that talent pool is on average much better suited for the job than your urban counterparts. Rural people by nature tend to be hardier, more self-reliant and more naturally skilled at soldiering. This is going to help you immensely for the next bits of organization. In fact, the old Russian word for "sniper" also meant, "close to the Earth," because the people they trained for the job generally came from rural or hunting backgrounds.

The next thing you are going to want to build is an infantry. At the same time, you'll be harnessing your local government to help you. Hey, wait a minute! Two paragraphs ago, didn't you tell us to exclude loose lips from the crew? Yes I did—for the Team and Team specifically. You should be able to tell your Team things you wouldn't tell a priest (including the address to the local boys school—zing!). Team is different. This isn't without precedent; we do this with host nation forces all the time. We might be best friends but some shit stays in the house. Now when we go outside of the house, we can have things we can say for public consumption.

In a rural Red county, you have an absolutely huge advantage that your government isn't that far disconnected from you. Your mayor isn't running around town smoking crack in a new Lincoln Navigator like Marion Barry. He is Bob down the street and odds are you know him. The same goes for all your city council nerds and the county Sheriff, all of whom are excellent assets.

Let's start with a general attitude and what you can get away with. If I went to a city council meeting in say, King County, Washington (Seattle) and I stood up and said, "This shit is out of control, I want to form a militia to sweep these Pantifa terrorists off the streets and I want the City Council to fund it!" What would happen? I would be escorted from the room, no doubt, and I might even go to jail for the hate crime of not addressing the tranny public works director by the right pronouns. Now how about if I try that same scenario in say, Salmon, Idaho? I'm probably gonna get applause from the audience and the city leadership just might surprise me. They might be like, "Fuck it, bro! You drill that militia in the town square every Sunday and we will be there with bells on!" Gaining the local Emergency Manager could be a huge win as well. The Emergency Manager already has access to all kinds of helpful tools like radios and maps. With a bit of prodding and some creativity, he can get a lot more.

The Federal Government and Department of Homeland Security have some really weird and really wasteful grant programs. All you need is someone smart enough to navigate the paperwork to get in on them. Out there in say, Bumfuck, Utah, does your town of 400 need military grade night vision goggles? Damn right they do. Hikers go missing all the time; sure would be helpful to be able to look for them at night, right class? How about one of those humongous armored trucks the military uses, the RG-33? Of course your town needs one, it's an all-terrain rescue vehicle. Just leave out the part about putting a snow plow on it to shove the commies off your streets if they show up.

Sheriffs are not a resource to ignore. As the highest elected law enforcement officer in the land, they carry a special kind of weight. They are also damn hard to get rid of by your local government should said local government not like them. In the last few years of crazy government overreach, we have seen some sheriffs step up as shining examples of the Founders' intent. We had deep Blue Virginia passing nutty gun laws from Richmond countered by County Sheriffs declaring 2nd Amendment sanctuary counties left and right. If you can recruit the local Sheriff to the cause, you have gained a very valuable ally.

The local Sheriff has access to some goodies too. With a pliable city council and some creativity, he has access to some really useful stuff like machine guns and grenade launchers. Maybe he can get a grant for training ammunition, since your department is poor and often has to dispatch mountain lions. DHS bought like a billion rounds of 40 Smith and Wesson two years ago. Lay hands on some if you can—consider it a tax refund. That isn't all the Sheriff can do. Law Enforcement has its own intelligence net accessible by anyone with the right credentials. Might it be helpful to know what are really the cutting edge tactics used by the current year domestic terrorists? I'm going with yes. Strength and composition information might very well be in there too. Not to mention the Sheriff can deputize anyone he damn well pleases, up to and including your entire town. That paints anything that comes next with at least a little bit of the color of the law.

Now since we just talked about the Sheriff, perhaps a little adjunct story time about cops is needed. I love the boys in blue. I've trained a shit ton of them in CQB and we always get along quite well, but 99.9% of the time, cops are always going to be cops. By that I mean they are going to default to their training and who they are until well after the situation has gone pear shaped and law no longer exists. I know this from experience. I was in a National Guard Special Forces Group before I was in an active duty one. National Guard SF has an extremely high ratio of cops compared to anything else I have seen. I was on a split team and of the seven of us, four were cops in real life, including the Captain. All of them were on their first tour, which also matters. The other three of us were raised by soldiers or, in my case, Marines, and we were not on our first tour. So like week one, off we go cruising down the highway in Iraq to do something stupid like meet the local rock farmers for tea or some shit. All of a sudden, here comes a white Corolla absolutely hauling ass on a trajectory to meet us head on—absolutely a no-no in this time and place. So one of the boys gives them a dose of 50 cal through the windshield, the car careens off the road and jumps a ditch, hub caps flying off, it was a borderline Hollywood car crash; smoke, dust, broken glass, the works. The Captain started freaking out: "Stop the truck, we have to check on them and write an incident report! I don't know... give them a reckless driving ticket, something." Our Team Sergeant is like, "No, we aren't. Sit down." So we get back to the base and the Captain is pissed. He starts yelling about how this isn't the Wild West and you can't just shoot at people, blah blah blah... because he has never seen a car bomb. One of the old hands says, "Hey motherfucker, actually it *is* the Wild West and the sooner you figure that out, the higher your chance of survival." That pretty much shut it down. Now to his credit, that Captain was as battle-hardened as it gets by the time that tour was over, as were my other cop teammates. My point is this: when we started, they were on a default setting of Police Officer with all the stuff that entails. That's great for some things but not for a war. Combat is not a police action and it will typically take some bad shit for them to unlearn being the Police. Now you may have Vic Mackey on the local force but it's not likely. So my advice is to keep the local 5-0 on your side, but not part of the inner circle.

Where were we? Oh yes, building an infantry. Your urban brethren can get away with having just a team of specialists; mostly because the best tactic they could use is to escape. That is not a luxury you can afford. You have to man the ramparts on which the wave of locusts breaks. You have to shatter the Commies' will to fight on the anvil of Grandpappy's Winchester, which means you need all the warm bodies with a gun you can muster. Don't interpret anything elitist from my use of the term "infantry" here. A professional Infantryman is a highly skilled individual with a depth and breadth of skills that are staggering. I was a Grunt and I think very highly of real USMC/Army Grunts. Not only do they carry an absolutely stunning amount of weight on the battlefield, but in recent conflicts at least, they do so with nowhere near the amount of glory they deserve. So perhaps a better description of what you need to build is an amateur infantry to go with your semi-pro team of specialists.

The difference is your infantry will be made out of people that don't have the time and dedication to devote to playing army for a situation that might not unfold. If you are training with your Team a minimum of once a week (preferably multiple times per week), your infantry formation is probably going to be lucky to muster once a month. People will get more interested and dedicated as things accelerate, so don't let a lack of commitment demoralize you. Also don't force the issue or you will just burn out your potential force. You can get away with this because your infantry won't actually need to learn that many skills. Like I said, a real Infantryman has to know all kinds of shit, but you don't have mortars, helicopters, a chemical or biological threat, a higher headquarters or a great many other things. Your force is going to be able to get by with just two skills from the offensive playbook and a dollop of defensive tactics. What if this goes the distance and you need the full arsenal of infantry tactics? That is beyond the scope of this book. I hope you have a real, seasoned Infantryman around to train you if that happens. I also recommend reading *The Last Hundred Yards* by H.J. Poole, *The Ranger Handbook, Attacks* by Erwin Rommel and *The USMC FMF 6-5.*

Hey Clay, this is sounding dangerously close to the dreaded *M-word*. Yes it does and it is high time we took that word back. I'm referring, of course, to "militia." I get it. For anyone that grew up in the time of Timothy McVeigh, militia is a very bad word. It conjurs up an image of some out of shape LARPing retard at the gun show talking about the black UN helicopters, etc. Meanwhile the only thing any of them ever managed to do in my lifetime was shoot a couple of Michigan State Troopers in the back and take over a trailer park in Texas for a couple of weeks—not exactly inspiring. This is exactly why we need to unfuck the connotation.

Our nation has a strong history of Militiamen from the Revolutionary War to the Indian Frontiers, and it brings a lot of benefits with it. Recently, once again in Virginia, we have seen some County Sheriffs actually blessing the freshly minted County Militia, which brings with it at least a hue of law. This may be very important as situations escalate. Also, it kind of paints the whole 2nd Amendment into a different light. Nobody has ever, to my knowledge, tried to argue that only the government can say who is and who isn't a militia. It might be fun just to form one and mount a legal challenge to the system if you have a pro-bono lawyer to lean on. A militia also makes people feel like they are part of something. Just slapping together an organization with a name does a lot for morale and recruiting. It doesn't matter a bit if half the people are just there for social hour. Hell, prior to 9/11 that is pretty much what the National Guard was. I saw 60 year old Privates in the West Virginia Guard who had been showing up for forty years instead of going to the Lions' Club. It instills at least a basic idea of being part of something bigger along with a teensy bit of military discipline. All wins, as far as I can tell. It doesn't really matter if you call it the Gem County Militia or the Placerville Civil Defense Force. If the M-word makes you cringe, pick something else; the principle is the same.

Unlike your small Team, this one you can advertise for. Put up fliers and slap a message on your town's Facebook page, because this formation you don't need to keep under wraps. In fact, the more open you are about it, probably the less nervous you are going to make your local ATF branch.

How else are you going to be able to short circuit negative optics on this? Easy, involve your local Sheriff's Department—provided you don't live in an absolutely dark Blue county. This once again plays to our advantage. Your Sheriff isn't snorting coke off a hooker's ass in a County-bought Lamborghini while trying to defend keeping the pension for some coward fuck that hid behind his squad car while a school massacre was happening. He is likely either someone you know or at least someone that is approachable. So go tell him what's up. Invite his deputies out to training. If you happen to have some real skills, not only will they benefit from it, but they will perhaps start seeing you as an asset. At the very least, they won't have to waste a bunch of time investigating if you are a whacko or not. If you put it out there on Main Street and include as many law abiding citizens as you can, a lot of mistrust is going to get put to bed.

What about the Feds? From a Federal standpoint, they aren't exactly fans of the Militia movement. I understand why, because pretty much all they have dealt with domestically for the last forty years are nutjobs and separatists; they kind of have a point. Expect to go on a list and expect an infiltrator or two. Am I really concerned about "being on a list?" No and neither should you. With the insane amount of data mining and NSA overreach via the Patriot Act, I assure you, you are already on a list. One off-color Kamala Harris meme too many, abnormal ammo purchases, maybe even just the wrong political opinions and you're on a list. This also isn't Soviet Russia (yet) so fuck the list. Do something, tough guy. What about the infiltration bit? Again, as long as you are coloring inside the lines, it's not a problem. Over the last five decades, the Feds have managed to infiltrate and destroy the KKK, Italian Mafia, several 1% Biker gangs and pretty much every other secret organization (somehow they can't do the same to Pantifa...*interesting*). So they are at least good at what they do. You can shut this down by not being a secret organization, keeping what needs to be compartmentalized compartmentalized and not doing illegal acts.

Remember the part where I said anyone talking about machine guns or bombs should be excommunicated and shunned? It goes double with a militia. You can also include Advocating Overthrow of the Government to that statement (check it, 18 US Code 2385). Anyone starts that shit, show them the boot. Look man, you aren't building a militia to march on Washington and storm the Capitol Building, you're building one to defend yourselves from hostile invaders the same as they would have back in the days of the Thirteen Colonies. Keep that mindset and quickly shut down any dipshit with a tinfoil hat and sedition on the mind.

So the ATF or FBI is going to possibly send either an undercover agent or an informant to the party—big deal, who cares? As long as you aren't doing anything incredibly stupid, it doesn't matter one bit. Besides, we have a bigger goal in mind. If every Red County in this country forms a militia, do they even have enough agents?

Okay, combat formations done. Do you need anything else? In the interest of not wasting manpower, you need to form an Auxiliary. An Auxiliary is a group of people that are sympathetic to your cause but are unwilling or unable to be directly involved. This might be a man that is too old to stand in the ranks, but can drive a truck like nobody's business and knows the mountains like the back of his hand. It could be purely financial. Some people may not want to really be in the mix but have enough of a vested interest in the town not burning to kick in some operational funds. Just don't go shake down Main Street like BLM is doing right now. "A Guerrilla must move among the people like a fish swims in the sea," as Mao said. Don't even think about asking for protection money. Not only will you lose the support of the people but local LE will come calling with a very unfriendly attitude. With that in mind, when it comes to financials, be very careful. I would go so far as to say let them come to you.

An Auxiliary can also include your intelligence net. We will cover that more in-depth later. It could be a local FFL that will let you buy a couple of pallets of blammo at distributor cost. It is pretty much anyone that is willing to help out in roles that don't include carrying a gun.

2   Lifeboat Rules

After *Concrete Jungle*, I got a lot of questions about incorporating women and children. Forgive me, I spent most of my life thinking about military things as a men-only club. So here we have a short chapter about including them in your plans.

Children, boys and girls, should absolutely be taught combat skills. Even if they don't need it this go around, it is handy to have in life. It also makes it a lot more palatable for everyone if your newfound hobby of shooting guns and walking around in the woods is a family affair. This is something you absolutely have to tailor to the age but don't forget this: in most of the world, a 13 year old boy is considered a fighting age male. It wasn't so long ago that this was true even in the United States. For that matter, one of my grandfathers lied about his age and enlisted in the Navy at 16 to fight in WW2. Your kids might need to do some fast growing up but their capabilities might surprise you. Start with tossing out the Xbox and giving them some responsibility, if you haven't already.

What about grown women? This is in no way a shock to most of you, but I am a bit of a sexist when it comes to fighting. I absolutely stand by the principle that women should not be on your front lines if at all possible... with a few caveats. First of all, of course your wife needs to know how to shoot. It's preposterous to think you are going to be on the farm blasting away at the Mongolian Horde with an AK-47 out the back door while the Missus is incapable of doing anything but knitting and policing strong language. Frontier women were not shy about slinging a carbine when necessary and you should adopt the same mentality. But that is not the same thing as setting them up in a blocking position with your infantry, by a damn sight.

However, there is one role that is perfect for women, and using them in this role will multiply your combat power immensely. Ladies, please stay with me as I explain. Shooting, particularly pistols and carbines, is strength and athleticism dependent. Especially if we aren't talking about slow, aimed fire at a tiny little bullseye. Combat shooting tends to be a cardio intensive event and because of that, no matter what the dude in your NRA class told you, women generally cannot compete with men. If I went to a regional USPSA match with all the big names, I could (and have) come in 50th place and still beat the female world champion. Same goes for 3 Gun, which is also a dynamic shoot and move sport. But there is one exception: Precision Rifle. Precise rifle fire is a bit of a different animal and in many contexts does not lean as much on athletic prowess. Therefore, women can and do hang with men even at the top levels. Google search the name 'Regina Milkovich.'

So there is a perfect niche for any women that really want to be involved. Designated Markswomen can be a force multiplier and are critical to some of the tactical situations we will be presenting in a few chapters. Just like everything else involving women, sniper rifles aren't cheap. At least if her gun costs more than yours you won't have to hear about it every time you start winning an argument.

Women also have a predisposition towards intelligence. I mean the gathering information kind, not the engineering kind (I bet that sentence alone earns at least a couple of one star ratings on Amazon. My sister was an Electrical and Mechanical Engineer, so eat me). Studies and life experience have shown that women talk more than men. Even in just raw words spoken per day, females dwarf males. So turn that gossip network into a group of spymasters. Women should be tasked to assess who may be a communist sympathizer. Sympathizers will be present in even the remotest of regions, so that's probably something you want to know. Are there visitors coming in? Does Aunt Jenny, the hippie from Portland, have the goods on a Terrorist Lives Matter plan to come "protest" your local Wal-Mart electronics department? There is a lot of information out there, you just have to look for it. Women can absolutely be a huge asset in this task.

3   Setting the Stage

Maybe I should have led with this point, but a lot of what this book entails isn't necessarily linear anyway (blame the traumatic brain injury and skip around as needed). It would probably help to talk about why so many things I talk about are a little bit vague and not tailored specifically to your exact situation. *Concrete Jungle* was simple in that regard. It was created for people that live in the big cities like New York, LA or Houston. That is easy because all cities are the same the world over. What works in one works in all of them. However, rural America covers terrain as varied as the forests of Maine and the Sonora Desert. Also, this volume kind of had to be for everyone else outside of the city. Time is not on our side and Purge Night isn't likely to wait on me to finish a fifteen book series covering every exact micro-climate. "Rural," for our purposes, means the obvious places like ranches and farms. It means the town of 200 in South Dakota that doesn't even show up on a GPS and is therefore impervious to an assault by marauding "protesters." It also covers any smaller city that is sufficiently isolated enough to have not been infected by the Blue Cancer. If you can walk out of it on foot in under an hour, it pretty much counts. Boise, Idaho; Billings, Montana and Amarillo, Texas, for example, all still fall under this umbrella. If the farmland within walking distance could sustain the population in calories, it probably counts.

As we hit on earlier, it works to your advantage that you tend to have fewer people but better raw material in terms of human capital. Your relationships with the local population are generally stronger. Not only are you more likely to actually know your neighbors, but statistically speaking you probably have long standing relationships with them. I could go back home, where I haven't lived in 23 years, and find 80% of the guys I went to high school with. Not to mention the network of other people that know me or my family from the generations that have lived there. The bugmen in the cities quite likely don't even know their direct neighbors. The culture, along with the transient nature of living in urban environments, doesn't create the same bonds. Your people are more likely to possess a variety of skills like running heavy equipment, hunting and four wheeling, which are all big bonuses.

However, your environment also possesses weaknesses. Even if it has better humans, you have a lot less of them. In many ways the upcoming contest for liberty is the ultimate showdown of r/K selection theory. Simplified, that means quantity vs. quality.

Your survival plan is much more dependent on logistics than your city brethren, which in many ways is like a cruel prank. You need more stuff and have the capacity to store more stuff, but the math says you are also likely to have less disposable income with which to acquire it. I'm not bagging on the rural areas, I'm just applying the obvious analysis from a US poverty/income map. Yes I know there are exceptions; welders, pipe fitters and plumbers may now have a laugh. I'm not talking about your individual financials,

I'm talking about the overall means of your base. Some will be people so poor they don't have a pot to piss in or a window to throw it out of. I am going to present a lot of things that sound expensive but remember, I'm just trying to cover the bases. Do not *ever* assume victory lies on material support only. It doesn't—but sometimes it does help.

If things get really bad, won't the US Military save the day? We will detail this in a later chapter, but the short answer is no, it isn't big enough. Depending on how this slides there just won't be enough of them. Right now, the military could absolutely shut these problems down. The areas actually in open revolt are small enough to contain. The National Guard could quell the riots and a single Task Force of SOF guys could eliminate the leadership and financial backing behind the revolt, but for a wide variety of political and legal reasons that won't happen. After this turns into a nationwide event, there's not a chance it *could* happen. A large-scale Blue Team vs. Red Team conflict becomes an absolutely *huge* peacekeeping operation if your desire is just to keep them from killing one another. Peacekeeping operations are much more manpower intensive than just breaking all the enemy's shit and going home. While we could very easily fight a land war against China or Russia, we could not occupy them in the long term. Iraq has a population one-sixth the size of the United States and it almost broke us militarily to occupy them for fifteen years, with probably 50 to 60% of their people largely sitting on the sidelines. In real terms, we have just about enough ground forces to occupy New York, LA and Atlanta at any one time. Start spreading that out across the country and it just doesn't work.

What can you do? Handle the business in your little corner of the world. Ten-thousand County Militias faithful to the Constitution make us stronger, not weaker. Even if this all goes away, you are doing your community and nation a service. If it doesn't go away and goes full up Civil War, should you be organized for that? Regional and State commands are beyond the scope of what you need to do right now. Not only do I have faith that those will arise organically if needed, but it's better to build bottom up than try and build top down. Besides, I was a Sergeant, not a Colonel; different skills for different needs. The best thing you can do is control your immediate area and make sure that you aren't a pile of spilt fuck if that day comes. Militias can easily form regiments and divisions with a dynamic leader. Military formations are essentially building blocks in that regard. Three squads make a platoon, three platoons make a company, three companies make a battalion, and so on and so forth with some overly complex Rube Goldberg officer shit thrown in to keep it from being too efficient.

Over the next couple of chapters I am going to walk you through some phases of what happens next in an insurgency. These phases differ from Pentagon approved source material because I'm not trying to write a doctoral thesis, I'm trying to simplify the steps on the road. Besides, I'm not qualified to write a doctoral thesis— I've actually been to combat—so don't @ me with some bullshit you learned at the War College, this book isn't meant to confuse new Lieutenants. These phases may also differ somewhat from the ones I put in *Concrete Jungle*; different situation, different words. Don't get wrapped around the axle with jargon; there is a lot of gray area between phases and it's a waste of time to try and figure out exactly where you sit. As we say on the pointy end of the stick, "there is no such thing as a low intensity conflict if you are the one being shot at." Like many things presented here, the phases are a guideline and not a hard and fast rule.

4   The Great Migration

If we were at the mall right now looking at the map, "Phase 1 – Refugees" would have the big red finger that says, "You are here." In August of 2020 at least, that is where we stand. While I could have also divided this into maybe Phase 0.5 refugees and Phase 1 refugees, we are consolidating. What exactly is a Phase 1 refugee? It is someone who has either flown the city because the peaceful protesters burned all their shit down and scared them off, or they're someone who has a second home in a rural region that they are hiding out in because peaceful protesters burned all their shit down and scared them off. This chapter will include advice for both you who are Phase 1 refugees and a little for those of us that have always had the sense not to live in some urban shithole.

Phase 1 refugees, first of all, it would help immensely to recognize that even if you personally are not one of the retards that voted for the policies that destroyed your natural home, you are still from there. You are going to be eyed with a healthy dose of suspicion until you prove not to be a liability. There are a lot of ways to prove this. For starters, if you haven't made the transition already, think about where you are going. I strongly recommend a town of at least a few thousand people, as it will make absorbing into the local landscape a lot easier. Towns of less than 400 are close knit in a way you wouldn't believe. You could be on the third generation in a place like that and still be thought of as the outsiders. A place a bit larger is going to have at least somewhat of a transient population and enough people that not everyone will instantly hate you. I also recommend that you pick a place more than one tank of fuel away from a Blue enclave (this will make more sense later, but distance is your friend).

Do not show up with #BLM, Refugees Welcome or Coexist stickers on your car. Not only is that going to instantly ID you as an enemy to your new Red county, but maybe a bit of self-reflection is in order as to why your native habitat turned into Mogadishu. To a lesser degree, get rid of your out of state plates and license ASAP. The less people that see you driving something from Commie-fornia the better. You will invariably be asked where you are from. I'm not saying to lie, because people will remember that and you will eventually make friends you'll have to be honest with, but saying you are from "Oregon" or "Minnesota" instead of "Portland" or "Minneapolis" is a much different thing. If pressed, it shows you are at least properly ashamed of where you fled.

Start dressing like the locals. A man bun and Birkenstocks might fit in great in San Francisco, but not so much in Dodge City, Kansas. Don't wear what you think rednecks dress like, wear what the locals actually wear. Anyone that has ever lived in a mountain town can spot the out of town hunters at a glance. They have the Gucci camo that still smells like the store and a carbon fiber chassis hunting gun in an exotic caliber with no scratches on it. Whereas the locals are in faded Real Tree with Carhartt jeans and a 30-06 older than they are. One trip to town and paying a bit of attention can keep you from sticking out like a sore thumb for the next year. This is an added expense but it's worth it.

This next piece of advice especially applies to the second home crew. If you are stocking up for the end times, bring the bulk of your supplies from out of town. This is for two reasons and the first is tactical. When COVID started, people all over Idaho and Montana had their personal shoppers buy up all manner of supplies. People that maybe step foot once a year in the state wiped out the stores via long range Visa card. They thought they were making themselves safe in case of a bug out, but what they actually did was make themselves loot boxes in case of a bug out. Look, those personal shoppers that maintain your property are locals. You might be keeping their kids in Huggies but you are not their best friend. If push actually comes to shove they will string you up for a can of beef-a-roni. Things are all cool and what not right now, but if the situation actually gets dicey, you ain't from there, son; you start holding the shortest straw. I don't care how good your nondisclosure agreement is either—people talk. How do you think I know about this? It will piss the locals off that you wiped the supplies out while flaunting your wealth. COVID didn't get people mad enough to string up the out of towners, but that possibility is always on the table. Especially in small towns, people don't respond well to flexing with the Benjamins. Avoid that when you can and leave some stuff on the shelf for everyone else.

Stocking up out of town is diametrically opposed to the next thing I am going to tell you. While it's true of bulk purchases, it isn't true for day to day shopping. Here, when you can, buy local. You being a good customer is a step towards turning the merchants in your favor and merchants are always going to be the first to turn. It not only transfers some dollars to a guy that runs a business in a rough economy, but it lets you interface with some humans from that region. Don't rush in and out like a mad man, chat 'em up a little bit. You will likely find the pace of life in a rural area shockingly slow, and it is. Sometimes the entire day's excitement is going to the store to buy a pack of smokes—I'm serious. So it is a thing to be relished, not rushed. Don't freak out if the cashier has a ten minute conversation with Jim while he buys a single six-pack. He has lived there for fifty years and has known her for thirty, you haven't.

Buying locally is good even if the local prices are inflated, and often they are. In a small place, you get a lot less turnover of goods and for perishables, a lot more waste. While the rent may be cheaper, it is still often a hardscrabble life running a grocery store in a small town. You will know you are starting to fit in when either they know your name and talk to you or you start getting the local discount. That last bit is for reals. I have lived in more than one place were the cash register had a 10% off button for literally anyone that was actually a local. I can't blame them a bit for soaking the weekend-only crew as a kind of tax. Welcome to anywhere with seasonal tourism.

This is also going to sound a bit contrary to the above, but hold both to be true and walk a thin line with it: if you have the means, overstock by design so that you have some rice and beans to hand out if things start getting thin. If not food, possibly some other goodies. If that sounds like a bribe, it is; sometimes that's how things work.

As a little aside, when I was working private security, I had a client that bought something like 47% of a little town all at once, then built a mansion on the hill. The locals fucking hated him. So to soothe tensions a little bit, he opened up a gaggle of empty lots as free parking areas. The tide turned; showing a bit of kindness in a weird situation can be enough to get you out of it. I'm not rich, you say? That is very much in the eye of the beholder. $150,000 yearly might make you a pauper in Manhattan, New York, but that is five times the annual median household income of Manhattan, Kansas. So if you just made a fortune selling your house on the coast at the right time, don't rub it in.

Won't overstocking by design also make me a loot box? If I have some to give away, I must have a lot more, right? It's a calculated risk. If things get really bad, you are going to see solutions we would never dream of in our spoiled day and age. Even if we are opposing Commies, you might see some collectivism have to start taking place to survive. We will talk about that later in logistics, but a little extra isn't going to hurt to have as either charity or barter. You might have a lot more means that other people.

Do you have a very valuable skill set? Let me tell you who no one is sad to see show up: doctors and nurses. If you are one, maybe offer some training to the local EMT crew or even host a monthly free clinic at the fire station. I know a veterinarian that lives with one foot in the city and one at his cabin in the mountains. Sewing up your dog costs about $500 in Salt Lake City but it costs a dinner in Backwoods, Utah. Do you write code for Google? Ask the local Emergency Manager if you can help him with his database systems. Hedge Fund Manager? In that case, probably just lie and say you blow dudes for a living.

But you say, "This is still America! What are some local yokels going to do?" Go for it, bro. Fly a Biden flag in the front yard and tell everyone how smart you are for being a marketing executive. You are correct, there is nothing in terms of legal means they can do to stop you. You may find out that the rules apply differently out in the sticks. I grew up in a place where the nearest Sheriff's Deputy was a 45 minute drive away in a best case scenario. That's if he was at the closest edge of his patrol route and not otherwise engaged. No kidding, we had to form a posse on more than one occasion to exterminate the packs of wild dogs people had dropped off on area ranches. I'm not that old, this was in the '80s and '90s. Plenty of Hollywood stars have bought a ranch in Montana and then bought a new radiator for their car every week until they decided to leave. Absolutely remember this: things are going downhill, obviously, and even the Hatfields and McCoys might unite to exterminate the Seattleites given the right set of circumstances. The best move is to stay off the target deck for the regional powers in case law and order completely breaks down.

What about you, long time Red County resident? Like I said, there's nothing in legal terms you can do to stop the inflow of refugees. In Boise, we have been dealing with the California invasion for ten years—get used to it. Still, there are some things you can do to build allies for the potential oncoming shooting match.

To some degree, numbers are going to matter, so if you can make converts it does pay to do so. First, realize that not everyone from the Blue Cancer states is a bad person. Northern California is full of rednecks that would easily be mistaken for natives of Alabama. Upstate New York is nothing like NYC and they hate NYC as much as the rest of us. Even if someone is from a Blue Metropolis, they may have seen the light recently. If they haven't fully, you can still ease them into our camp. As I mentioned about skills, if you make friends with the newbies you might find they have something to teach you as well. Showing someone the ropes and just how good we have it out here can go a long way towards conversion. If this turns into an all hands on deck shooting war, you want all the help you can get.

DISCLAIMER

Nothing from this point forward should be taken as legal advice. For that matter, nothing I say to anyone *ever* should be taken as legal advice. I was a warfighter, not a lawyer. My understanding of the law is at best half-assed and perhaps even quarter-assed. A lot of what I am about to tell you is absolutely not legal in the United States and quite possibly not legal if you believe in the Law of Land Warfare or International Conventions on Armed Conflict. I am not telling you what to do. I am telling you what some options may be—in Minecraft. *Caveat Emptor.*

Also, it's my book so I'm going to take a second and say I hate lawyers. The beginning of our failing as a nation is when we started letting limp-wristed, soy boy, over-educated cucks interpret the Founders' intent. If I woke up tomorrow to discover all the lawyers on Earth had been shot into the sun, friends and family that are attorneys included, I couldn't possibly stop smiling for weeks. They are a huge part of the reason we are in this fucking mess.

John, Kurt Schlichter and the dude that represented that smirking kid against CNN get a waiver.

5 Bantu on the Warpath

" It is criminal to teach a man not to defend himself when he is the constant victim of brutal attacks"- Malcom X, 1965

In this chapter we are going to talk about Phase 1 tactics, which require a little bit of a history lesson to understand the other side. Bear with me for a few minutes. I also need you to recognize something right now that is going to be uncomfortable for a lot of you: we are getting our asses kicked. Writing this in August of 2020, it has been like ninety days of lopsided beatings for our team with a very few bright spots of hope. For example, that fat Pantifa retard in Austin that tried to scare someone in a car with his AK-47 and in turn got blasted by a dude with a hand cannon; hats off, brother— way to win one for the good guys.

Getting housed is not entirely unexpected, nor our fault. We are facing an enemy that has been plotting for sixty years waiting on just this moment. They are well entrenched with complete top cover from both the mainstream media and often the State. They are also fighting with a style of warfare that is completely foreign to most of us.

What I see in these riots and street fights is tribal warfare with all the hallmarks of it that one would expect. Rural America (I would contend *all* of America up to about 1955) has absolutely no clue how to process tribal warfare because our people don't fight like that. Tribal warfare from Africa or pre-Conquistador South and Central America looks very similar, and was probably similar the world over at one time. Both sides line up on the field, preferably in scary costumes, then they make loud noises by beating on shields or whatever. Some ritual dance moves to intimidate the other side might happen, some projectile weapons may be exchanged (often at a range where they have no chance of hurting anyone) and then 99 times out of 100 both sides go home and declare victory. Deaths are rare. Real close range blood baths do happen but not often. When they do happen it's almost like the shit talk just got out of hand.

If you think I'm kidding, even the Aztecs, the feared superpower of pre-European Central America, didn't get far past that. They often had armies mass and then had one on one fights. You might win your fight and you go home with the losing Aztec dude as a prisoner. However, a hundred of your guys also lost so they go home as Aztec prisoners while very much alive, which is how they fueled the human sacrifice part of their religion. That sounds insane, right? Even the mighty Greek Phalanx, at least when fighting other Greeks, was more of a pushing match than a battle. Some soldiers might die, sure, but it was never a slaughter unless one side broke and ran. This says a lot about both the method of war and the human instinct to pounce if someone or something is fleeing.

All of which is diametrically opposed to the way that Europeans, Asians and certainly the hard-ass bastards of the Eurasian Steppe conducted warfare. In Europe, we can probably look to the Ancient Romans as the ones that changed things. The best way to describe a Roman Legion is to call them mass produced Spartans. When a Legion came to town, it didn't waste time playing "no, you hit me first" while impotently shoving back and forth; they would just kill your ass. Then they met worthy adversaries in German barbarians, Celts and others that also always played for keeps. By the time of Napoleon, if a European army took the field, it was going to fight. Americans obviously descended from that same school of thought and then turned it up to eleven on the new continent. We have no idea how, perhaps, Native Americans fought each other, but we do know that at least against the American invaders they played to win—not by making noises while trying to look hard.

My point here is we have no cultural frame of reference for tribal style conflict. Americans were actually known for a very long time the world over as doers, not talkers. Back on the frontier, you didn't talk shit because you probably would have to back it up. You might just get shot for being a mouthy little bitch. Conservative Americans also generally don't protest in the streets. Not only do we have day jobs, but the idea of marching around with cute slogans on signs just isn't us. We flirted with the idea a bit in the Tea Party days, but even that was a tiny minority.

Not only are we facing a completely foreign method of tribal warfare, but it is a highly evolved version thereof that's been brilliant so far in execution. Most of that mass is made up of low IQ people that really think they are changing something with chants and dances. Intermixed with them are terrorist elements and opportunistic looters. The mass hangs on because it looks like not only are they on the winning team, but they don't actually have to do anything. They just get to be close to the action and cheer like they're in box seats at a foosball game. But their numbers provide cover for the bad apples and it becomes a self sustaining organism. Carrot and stick, wrapped up in one package.

Yes, this is actually dangerous—because it is working. They are gaining ground and terrorizing middle America without ever having to step foot in it. The optics look really bad and that is demoralizing to our fence-sitters. This is an example of 4th Generation Warfare and it stands just as much chance of overthrowing our government if left unchecked as a shooting war would. For further reading, I would encourage you to check out both Color Revolutions in general and *The New Rules of War* by Sean McFate. McFate and I might disagree on some minor points but his book is absolutely excellent for understanding 4th Gen War.

This is where things went totally off the rails. I had written another 20 pages of outstanding phase 1 tactics, which in my opinion is exactly what we should do. Then I submitted this chapter for review, and the legal team said absolutely not. Which left me with three options. 1- Publish it anyway, and consequences be damned. Which would've no doubt gotten us pulled from Amazon, and you wouldn't have a book. Plus, I would spend the next two years defending myself from the Soros machine lawsuits.

Option 2- I could have watered this section down to the point it was unrecognizable and given you a bunch of feel good fluff. That would be pointless. The idea here is to save your ass and chucking in a bunch of nonsense filler wastes both your and my time.

Option 3- What I am going to do. Given how much the attorney's pitched a fit, it is best to just skip this part. You can think, and I have a lot of important things to share besides specific tactics. Remember when I said stay out of the streets? This is me taking my own advice. Especially when I can point you to open source materials that pretty much say the same thing I would, if you dig a little and use your noggin. But what about my First Amendment? This is more lawyer cuckery, but it's true. The magic paper is absolutely not going to defend you. And you had best stop thinking it will. I hate that this is the state of things in 2020, but as we say in the business. Shit in one hand and hope in the other. See which one fills up faster.

Further reading- Rex Applegate (the father of a great many things) Riot Control: Material and Techniques.

6   Trail of Tears

Moving on from Phase 1, we will now enter Phase 2. We have to set the stage a little bit about how things evolve so it makes sense to combine refugee and tactical considerations into one chapter. The first item on the agenda is to think about how enemy tactics will change. The whole fiasco could shut down after a few ass whippings Phase 1 style, but I wouldn't bank on it. Outside of a *very* strong Federal response to the embers of insurrection in Phase 1, which doesn't seem to be on the menu, the situation will escalate. Commies, while they have 57 genders and can't figure out which bathroom to use, are not stupid. It is a common misconception by those who have never been to war to assume your opposition is stupid. It wasn't true in Afghanistan or Iraq and it won't be true here. They will adapt and evolve. As my mentor Col. Tonn was fond of saying, "Never forget that your enemy is human and capable of thinking just like you."

As for how this is going to go, I can predict, as well as have seen on a limited scale, Pantifa absolutely getting its ass handed to it when it tries Portland tactics against Red America. Unfortunately, like we briefed, the vast majority of them will survive those encounters. The next step for them is to adopt traditional Left Wing tactics. Bombings are a strong suit for them. The fact Bill Ayers is still walking this Earth is a sin against God and man. Bombs are like the unskilled man's sniper rifle. They're an easy tactic and a traditional favorite after Lefties start getting their asses handed to them in gunfights. They don't care about collateral damage, so they start chucking bombs out willy-nilly. Targeted assassination of our political leaders is another. The rhetoric is already there. We are one baby step away from "People's Courts" and fatwahs with death sentences handed out by a tribunal of Social Justice Warriors. Flash mobs are a favorite of the Left, though in this phase it will be guns and edged weapons, not just beating and looting. In areas that don't resist, it wouldn't be out of character for people to just be dragged from their homes and hung from lampposts, or put up against the wall and shot (not exactly without Commie precedent).

We will also likely see something akin to small scale raids for either resources or just to inflict damage. These will be driven not just by ideology (get the Red Team) but by necessity. As the city situation gets worse, it isn't unthinkable they will be cut off logistically. Already during COVID, truckers publicly stated they might not make deliveries to NYC. This was due to fear of hunger mobs, not the disease. Every truck driver in this country knows the name Reginald Denny and they aren't stupid. We have already seen Amazon and FedEx trucks looted and burned just during Phase 1 riots. Only an idiot would drive a McDonalds resupply truck into urban America during Phase 2. Expect mobs to not only show up to potentially do an overgrown drive-by, but to take shit besides your TVs.

Phase 2 is that gray area between civilized society and war. You probably won't be able to get away with just blasting anyone with out of state plates, but you are also going to have to be a bit more flexible with what you are willing to do. Legalities are still a concern because even at full up Phase 2, the situation could back down. As well, most people are slower to adapt than you might think. Idealism runs high, especially in law enforcement communities. This is yet another reason that cops aren't soldiers and soldiers aren't cops. It's also a big part of why terrorism should never be treated as a law enforcement issue, though it often is, even in overseas adventures.

As a little aside here, we saw all the time in Special Forces how the normal citizens' minds refuse to mold in a situation like this, at least initially. You'd get some new pimple faced college boy as a Captain. If it's late in the war, he actually has a little bit of combat time as an Infantry/Armor Company Commander, but combat time is a lot different, in this war at least, for a Company Commander versus some hard-nosed squad leader. So your Captain is still full of all the ideals they beat into him at West Point or the Citadel: *bad guys always have a uniform on, they are coming right for me and I had no choice but to shoot them! Of course, I'll get a Purple Heart (just a flesh wound, nothing serious) and a medal for Valor. Later, after I make General (with a hot secretary, no doubt) and retire, I'll get that six figure book deal where I talk about making hard choices and Army values and how awesome the Academy made me...* And he is in charge of eleven pipe hitters that have been playing whack-a-mole with the same assholes for the last five tours. The new Captain is out of his depth. He keeps asking why you shot that guy, or telling you not to kill the guy on a cell phone because he doesn't understand that if you don't, you are going to start taking really, really precise mortar fire in about two minutes. He keeps spazzing out and the Team Sergeant has to keep slapping him around... until something really bad happens. Next thing you know, he is ready to justify dropping JDAMs on the local bazaar if he just *thinks* weapons might be present. You can actually see the change in an officer's eyes the first time he loses someone under his command, up close and personal. Idealism dies and the truth of human nature fills its place.

This is also one of the reasons that combat veterans and formations led by combat veterans will be so dangerous early in the coming conflict. Our threshold for savagery is already beyond description. We have had all the ingrained and evolved humankind violence limiters beaten out of us already. We have no morality to overcome in terms of blowing someone's fucking head off, preferably while they are sitting at their dining room table with no chance to return the favor… Okay, soap box rant over. The long and short is you will have some fuckery to overcome. You can't just start dropping artillery on Oakland but you also can't just sit around with the hickory stick or your dick in your hand from Phase 1, that ship has sailed.

Let's first talk about Phase 2 refugees. Unlike Phase 1 mass migration, Phase 2 is unlikely to show up with a Uhaul truck and a place to live. This will actually be your first wave of true refugees, some of them showing up with just the shirt on their back. They will be entirely dependent on the local community for a roof over their heads and will start to strain your supply lines. This is going to happen two ways. The first will be the smart people that saw life in the city as unsustainable and got out of Dodge. Believe it or not, in August of 2020 this is already happening. Every campground in Idaho and Montana is packed full with a huge percentage of those people looking for a place to rent or buy. This is a frightening indicator of how bad things are already, but a fact nonetheless.

Stuff crammed in storage lockers; these poor bastards are holding it down at the KOA waiting on the dust to settle. While this is initially a boom for business, with just a little increase in numbers it starts to really affect food, fuel, hard goods, etc.

It can also overwhelm local infrastructure. Talk to anyone that lived in the boom towns of South Dakota when oil started flowing. There were so many imported workers that in some cases it was more than the existing sewer and water systems could handle. At least under normal conditions, some of that could be fixed with emergency upgrade funding. We likely don't have that kind of time.

As law and order are still in place (kind of) for this phase, your options are pretty limited. This is a local government issue and your local government may not have the balls to handle it. You can go a couple of ways, just keep in mind that no matter what you choose there are a finite number of refugees you can take in without collapsing your ecosystem. Option one is to do what you can for these poor bastards. A common occurrence out West when snow closes the roads and the hotels can't handle the volume is to open up the school as a temporary shelter. There are a lot of publicly owned facilities that you can use for housing in a pinch, with the need rather tied to the climate. It also isn't without precedent for the local government to start administering hobo camps. As recently as the Great Depression this was a thing. Are you ready for some decidedly unsexy talk? Good.

[Let me keep your attention... Max Commando realized it was the part of the story when he needed to fight the largest bad guy in hand-to-hand combat. He threw down his gun and turned to face his comically muscled, vaguely Eastern European opponent. "I also am trained in Krav McJitsu," he said. Hey, camp administration is fucking lame for a survival book, I get it, but it doesn't mean it isn't going to happen...]

The number one thing you need to know about camps is that hygiene is king. If you start cramming people together in shanty towns by slapping shelters together willy-nilly, outbreaks of disease are going to run like wildfire. They won't just affect the refugees, that shit (in some cases literally) will spill over and ruin your day. To use the technical terminology, it will fuck *all* your shit up. You must address this early and stay on top of it. Good resources exist to help you out with this from FEMA manuals to UN literature. If you get the UN manuals, please skip over the 'rape and sexual extortion for beans' parts—fucking animals. The base idea is that you need to keep things neat and tidy as well as keep the people as clean as possible. A civil engineer is a good dude to put in charge of this, though even a Boy Scout Master is going to do a fine job.

You can tell a lot about how well a camp is running by the basic layout. Does it have wide avenues that resemble streets and blocks or is it a clusterfuck of guy lines and plastic tarps just slapped up? Planning for this up front is going to pay off in spades. Rows and columns not only contribute to appearance and refugee morale but also in logistics. If things look neat it is easier for the inhabitants to take pride in keeping it that way. That actually does matter; these poor bastards need something to hang on to, and keeping their extremely humble lodging in order might just be what keeps them from tipping over the edge. Second, it makes it easier to administrate. If you have blocks with numbers, you can find that dude you need to find in a hurry, survey at will, and keep an accurate count. It also makes it possible to evacuate in the event of a fire (the bane of all such camps) and to keep said fire from spreading out of control. It also eases things like garbage removal and organizing work details.

Community latrines are going to be a big part of this, so you need to think about that ahead of time. Pee-pee and poo-poo are not your friends but they happen every day. You have to keep people from pissing in the street as your number one fight against disease. Be it slit trenches or poop buckets, you gotta plan for it. Showers, too; even if you can only get your refugees one shower per week, that is going to help immensely. Warm water would be a huge bonus if you can swing it.

Community kitchens are also going to be in order. It is not only inefficient to have individual cooking in the camp, but it also increases the risk of fire. Besides, these people aren't going to have a lot of resources. Not only do they likely not have any money for food, but it is more wasteful to try and feed each family separately. This all sounds pretty savage—and it is—but we are all going to spend a lot of nights cold and hungry before this is over, trust me. The best thing you can do right now is prepare your mind for that eventuality.

Phase 2 refugees aren't all going to be strangers either. You are likely to be asked for safe harbor by extended family members, old Army buddies, etc. You aren't going to treat them like randos, obviously, but this also isn't a vacation, so you need to handle things a bit differently. The good thing here is this group is likely to show up with some resources in tow. They also may have been burned out and left with nothing, but the odds are good they are coming early and bringing some stuff with them. The first thing you want to establish before you agree to take them in is that this likely isn't temporary. They may believe it is and they may tell you it is, but in situations like this, temporary is all but guaranteed to become permanent. So make damn sure they bring all the supplies they can. If you can coordinate it, pre-staging of supplies by your guests is a really good idea. It's not exactly an original thought; I can easily credit James Wesley Rawles and his book *Patriots* with that. We will hit Rawles again in some later chapters as he is arguably the father of the modern survival movement. While I heartily disagree with some of his output, he is pretty well versed in a great many things. Both his fiction and non fiction are recommended, but read his fiction with a large grain of salt.

As your friends, family or whoever show up as Phase 2 refugees, it is best to set them up in for semi-permanent living. If the situation escalates this far it isn't likely to get better overnight. Have you ever had guests living in your house for an extended period of time? I have and it doesn't take long for them to start to get annoying, no matter how cool they are. Next thing you know you are tripping over each other, homeboy is sitting in your favorite chair, kids are fighting over toys... For long term mental health and stability, it just isn't great. Therefore, I recommend that if at all possible, you create some other kind of space for your castaways. If you live in a mansion on the hill, maybe you can just give them a wing of the palace, but that isn't real life for most of us. So you gotta think outside the box a little bit. A garage conversion isn't bad, but it is almost the same thing as them being right in your house. If you have any kind of outbuildings like a barn, that is what I would use.

Now that sounds kind of mean in our spoiled, luxurious day and age, but it is actually going to be better for everyone. First of all, it keeps the riff-raff out. No one is going to show up to live in the barn if things aren't actually dire. This way you aren't burning up supplies and spousal goodwill every time Pantifa throws a Molotov in Portland. In a 'boy who cried wolf' type of way, your guests won't evacuate until they actually need to. Second, there's the mental health benefit of not losing all your personal space. Third, it gives some pride of ownership to the people you're sheltering. As a man, you never want to be a freeloader. It is actually bad for us mentally; especially bad for the kinds of people you are likely to be taking in. Having your own space that you've earned, even if it's meager, is worth nearly any price.

While most Americans today are accustomed to relative opulence compared to our ancestors, a barn or shed space doesn't have to be an unthinkable solution. Hunting cabins around these parts are quite spartan and that is a preferred living solution for many men for weeks out of the year. Hell, tiny houses are routinely made out of sheds and that is a lifestyle choice more popular by the day. You don't want to spend a fortune creating the Taj Mahal when that money could have been better spent on supplies, but you can make something livable pretty cheap. An old school wood stove can often be had at a yard sale or from a classified ad which solves a lot of problems. Even a tiny camping version will do a fantastic job in a small space.

Speaking of camping, a yurt or a wall tent can solve this problem pretty well too. You might not think it but a yurt especially will take a snow and wind load like you wouldn't believe. A surplus military tent, provided you aren't too lazy to scrape the snow off before it builds up, will work in absolutely any environment. With a pallet and plywood floor it makes a more cozy living space than our spoiled ass modern Yankee standards would imply.

Maintaining a camp is a great option, as it gives your guests something to do. They get the mental health boost not only of having a home, but of daily improvements in their position. Long periods of boredom and brokenness will precede Phase 3. It can fill a lot of time learning how to make a log chair, bartering some chicken eggs off for some personal touches via the local economy, and the daily cleaning and maintenance such a living space requires.

The basic gist here is to start thinking like a poor person if you don't already. Cheap travel trailers that maybe aren't road worthy anymore also make a great solution if you are prepared to do a little work. I've seen entire families winter over multiple years in Canada in nothing more than a travel trailer with some hay bales for exterior insulation. It can be done and it doesn't mean you have to suffer in the process. Toss some overhead cover on that bad Johnson and you are in hog heaven.

Odds are decent your visitors won't be remote working during this process. COVID has definitely taught us that while that may work in some career fields, it definitely doesn't work for all. Not to mention, we can expect the economy to crater at some point during or before Phase 2, so it is also a good idea to share some chores with the new guys. This has a couple of benefits. One, you aren't going to get bitter if you are still going to work everyday while ya boy sits in the Laz-E Boy cracking cold ones. Two, as mentioned, no man likes the feeling of being a freeloading piece of shit. It is going to be better for everyone if the transients have some stuff to do. I think, maybe, women are the same way (if I actually understood how women think and act, I would be writing an entirely different book and I would probably be rich, so let's go with a blind assumption here). These tasks can be actual needs or, to some degree, just make work. That also doesn't sound nice but the military has proven it is better to have something stupid to do than nothing to do. However, I very seriously doubt you will be short on things to do. Chopping wood, digging defenses, minding the chicken coop, none of what is coming will be easy. You could also reasonably put your new manpower on security detail for part of the night, not only to become accustomed to doing so, but as a simple and productive task.

Much like the community kitchen mentioned for the hobo camps at the beginning of this chapter, you will probably want to do the same in your home. Not only does it conserve resources like fuel, but it is likely to be a necessity anyway. You will have to start rationing at some point in this conflict; no one is getting out of this fat and happy. Breaking bread together is also a long standing method of human bonding and meal times are great social times. So if you are housing an entire separate family unit or couple, they can help out here too. It may be an initial cause of consternation to ask your spouse to share her kitchen, but letting the other team handle meal prep on a rotation basis is a good idea. It not only balances the workload a bit but it makes them feel more at home.

We solved this pretty easily when I was in the Special Forces Qualification Course, albeit we were all bachelors at the time. I had a house with like five roommates that we called the FOB. After about a week of Cheerios and beer can pyramids, we decided that we didn't want to live like savages (well, at least not *total* savages). So we devised a system that was pretty simple. We had a white board with all the shit that had to happen at the house during a week as tasks. Jobs were assigned on Sunday at the weekly FOB meeting. Monday through Friday, every dude got assigned dinner prep one night. If you cooked, the next day you had clean up duty; a good system since we all had homework and Army shit to do as well. Doing one task cost you an hour or so instead of three or four hours in one day. That FOB ran for like seven years; long after all the original members graduated and left or got married or whatever. I know because my name was still on the lease—they had to come find me to shut it down.

The point is, you don't need to give your guests like eight hours of manual labor per day to make them feel like part of the team. Don't put them out there picking cotton and singing songs like 1920s share croppers, but don't let them get a total free ride either. It's bad for everyone. I strongly recommend a viewing of an episode of the cartoon *The Boondocks* called, "The Invasion of the Katrinians" for reference.

Moving on, let's now talk in depth a bit about Phase 2 tactics. Phase 2 exists in the gray area between US law being enforced and outright insurgency. That is a pretty broad range of what can happen to determine how you should react. Let's put it in easy to understand terms.

What happens if you ambush and slaughter a convoy of Pantifa Goons in Phase 3 open combat? Bottle Caps of Valor all around (*Calvin and Hobbes, Bill Watterson, Aug 20 1993*) and you don't have to buy drinks for a week or so. What if you do the same thing in Phase 1? You go to 'pound me in the ass' prison for premeditated murder and spend the opening months of the jihad behind bars. You should've and could've just called the cops. In Phase 1, you are still paying them to handle things like rabble-rousers and arsonists. Now how about in Phase 2? Good question— it is very situation dependent. It's shitty but I don't have a good answer for every scenario and neither does anyone else. All of us that spent time in the Balkans and/or the GWOT, depending on the year and the level of cuckoldry of your first line command up through Commanding General displayed, can relate. It's very much a judgment issue and you will be Monday morning quarterbacked by dipshits that weren't on scene. Doubly so since we live in the time of everything recorded on video, often without context. Between law and war there are a lot of ways to get hung—get used to it. That being said, it's generally best to err on the side of legal means and ways. I hate it as much as you do, but this is the weak sister world we live in. Hope is not an operational strategy and wishes aren't tactics, but you can still stack the deck in your favor and lay the groundwork for what comes next.

Let's look at a likely Phase 2 Blue tactic: the raid, to either cause damage to you or steal your supplies. For once, the military definition is pretty useful: "A raid is an operation, usually small scale, involving a swift penetration of hostile territory to secure information, confuse the enemy or to destroy his installations. It ends with a planned withdrawal upon completion of the assigned mission." Basically, a short attack not intended to hold any ground. A home invasion but scaled up a bit. How can you counter such a thing while staying on the side of the line that doesn't involve landmines or a pre-emptive strike on a staging area?

One very useful idea is to start controlling access to your town or space. This is much easier to do with the support and endorsement of local governance. From a purely legal standpoint, can you put up a checkpoint on each end of the road going through your town? I didn't go to Harvard but I can pretty safely say no. But how about your County Sheriff? Well, precedent would say yes. It can be a 24 hour manned DUI checkpoint perhaps, or martial law can be declared for your county, which gives all sorts of new powers to the local LE. Maybe that checkpoint has one real deputy and a gaggle of "reserve" deputies put on the books because of a crisis. If that road happens to be a state or Federal Highway, this is probably not likely to stand up to a court challenge, but even an injunction by the ACLU is going to take time. If your County Sheriff has a set of balls on him, someone would still have to divert State or Federal forces to make him stop. Part of the play here is to time things like this so that higher level resources can't be spared to oppose you.

Restricting travel movements sounds pretty un-American and directly contrary to what we are fighting for. I get that. As a 1st Amendment and freedom purist, I am 100% with you. It is distasteful for me to even contemplate this, much less tell you it needs to be done, but I am also a realist. The Magic Paper, aka the Constitution, isn't going to protect you. Over the last 100 years, it has actually succeeded in protecting exactly jack and shit. There may be time to fix this later but there will not be a later if you lose. It is foolish and suicidal to try and play by the rules when one side has already gone full up "by any means necessary." That is an actual slogan as well as the name of an organization on the Left, and they mean it. How else can you explain the fact that BLM and Pantifa are using blatant terrorism in the streets while politically telling us it will stop if we just submit to Joe and the Hoe? Once again, this is reality giving you a hard slap on the keister. It doesn't matter if you like it, facts don't give a shit about your feelings.

What else can you do to prevent shenanigans in your AO? Defense sucks and it's no way to win a conflict, but a lot of what you need to do in this phase is defensive in nature. Along with the DUI checkpoints, you might start security patrols, particularly after dark. We will cover patrolling operations in depth later in the book, but for now let's just call it a couple goons on a walkabout. Can you get away with this? Well, the entire structure of neighborhood watch associations says yes. Yours just happens to be packing some heat, provided you live in a jurisdiction where that's legal.

If you have enough resources, two to three goons covering a shift of a few hours can be a powerful deterrent to infiltration. It's enough firepower to at least make them think twice and buy your team enough time to wake up and react. It's enough manpower so as to not be easily overwhelmed and killed by a quiet sneak attack. Sending more than one person also helps alleviate potential tomfoolery by your own guys. One man, alone, can easily be accused or guilty of things like window peeping, "liberating" outside storage or checking unlocked cars for loose change. A team of people is much less likely to give into such temptations.

In order to make this work, it is best to have it be known by the locals that you are doing so. Once again, I recommend some easily identifiable clothing like neon green construction shirts from day one. This is one of the limited times that being readily identifiable is more important than camouflage for tactical reasons.

First, if a gunfight does kick off, the responding reinforcements can tell which side is which pretty easily. Second, it lets the citizenry tell at a glance that you are supposed to be poking around on the side streets in the middle of the night. This keeps them from calling the local five-oh and negating any good work you did by chewing up other resources to investigate your own. Third, at least initially, it is unlikely to be duplicated by the enemy. Even if they do later, the odds of someone not noticing two patrols or the two not bumping into one another are pretty slim.

I'm going to add a little real world experience to this one. One time at band camp, my Task Force turned the corner into some shithole little neighborhood and immediately ran into a couple dozen Iraqis out in the street and armed to the teeth. The only thing that kept us from blazing them with a mini gun was the fact they were all wearing US Army issued neon PT belts. Now we had no idea what in the fuck was going on, but just the sheer absurdity of the situation kept us from opening fire, surprised as we were. The 'terps did some jibber-jabber, defused the situation and we went down the street to do whatever it was we came to do. It was a good thing we did, because those PT belts represent the uniform of the Sunni Awakening and we would have melted down the 4th Infantry Division's freshly minted militia. Methinks Mr. Petraeus would have been upset with us. Now we had no idea what was going on driving into that and were in a known hostile region. Sans yellow glow in the dark belts, it would have been weapons free instantly. My point is that sometimes sticking out is actually a good idea.

How else can you enhance this process? Coordinate with local LE if possible. You could even do your shift changes at the

Department so they know you are around. If your cops can spare a radio to pass around to the neighborhood watch, that is also hugely helpful. An electric golf cart would be the ideal neighborhood watch add on. While extremely limited in range, it does offer some big benefits. You will be able to cover more ground and the cart goes faster in a pinch than most people can run, at least for longer distances. Because they are near silent, your dudes don't lose a lot of either awareness nor sneakiness. Also any soldier knows that walking the same patch of streets night after night gets very boring and kind of tiring. You put a bunch of out of shape bros on foot patrol and you will be out of volunteers inside of a week.

That covers your short range needs. If you have the manpower to support it, and certainly as the tactical need escalates, you can apply the same mentality to mechanized patrols around your area. As in, use a car or truck to get further out from home base. The further out you intercept an enemy force, the less your odds of taking collateral damage to your stuff or bystanders. This would not only be the lesser known roads and paths to your town, but around the farm and ranch "outposts" that we will cover later. The same principle applies of making yourself easy to ID. I would stay away from the blue and red lights, but something as simple as a yellow or green strobe light on the roof can be a good far-away recognition symbol. Over time, any outposts will be able to pick up the sound of your particular patrol rig, especially if your group buys one for this purpose. That is a good thing because as things get worse, you are going to want to stop patrolling with lights.

During this phase, you probably want to toss some spotlights in those rigs too. You know, the kind of spotlights that I am absolutely positive none of you good ol' boys own for jackrabbits. A lot of things you might miss from the road, a spotlight can pick up to the flanks. Another reason to have multiple people in a vehicle even for a low threat security patrol is the driver *always* just drives. The other one or two monkeys can spotlight or shoot as the situation dictates.

This is a big step but at this point you want to get the local citizenry onboard with clearcutting around anything you need to secure. Ask any Vietnam vet, this is like step one of establishing a firebase. If you have to get in a gunfight, distance is your friend. If vegetation or trees comes right up to the edge of your town, it is nearly impossible to stop infiltration. Cut that back 100 yards and any opposing forces have their work cut out for them to try and crawl their happy asses in. In a wooded area, this is a huge undertaking. Out on the plains, it might be as simple as a couple of laps with the brush hog. Because of all the land ownership undoubtedly involved, this will not be a simple undertaking, but getting it done will save a lot of blood and sweat later when it *has* to be done.

The same goes for identifying and fixing concealed routes into town that are foot accessible. In military terms, we would call low spots on the ground that offer protection from observation and direct fire "defilade." If we had some of that outside of an outpost, we would occasionally lob grenades or mortar rounds into it just in case. You don't have any indirect fire weapons so that isn't an option, but you can often fix them up with some razor wire or broken glass to discourage infiltration. This isn't foolproof by any means. Another military maxim that is true is that an obstacle is only an obstacle if it is covered by fire. This means that if you don't have a gun covering that razor wire 24/7 it isn't much more than a feel good measure. In this phase of the conflict though, it is probably good enough. It also gives your roving patrols something to keep an eye on. The Border Patrol is notoriously good at spotting footprints and clothing threads on wire, even at high rates of speed. If you routinely check on your defilade areas, you will at least know when someone has been through them.

Lastly for Phase 2, you should be all about further preparation. You will likely have more people showing up to volunteer and in general getting a lot more nervous. Things can still back down at this point so don't put the chips all in before you have to. They can also escalate to full up Phase 3, in which case the brakes are out and we are going for a ride.

7   Highway to Hell

In order to get to Phase 3, we are talking about some absolutely crazy shit. Do you remember when that militia went all crazy in Texas in the '90s and took over a trailer park, resulting in a months long standoff? Or the CHAZ autonomous zone from just a little while back? Lakota tribesmen seizing the town of Wounded Knee in 1973, resulting in a standoff lasting 71 days? All of those are still law enforcement sized problems, Federal Law Enforcement at the worst. Compared to what would constitute Phase 3, those are chump change. In order to pass from Phase 2 to Phase 3, we are talking about absolutely off the rails, way outside what normal people consider possible, dogs and cats living together, complete pandemonium tier events that would need to happen. Still, the possibility exists and I for one would rather be prepared for space alien zombies than surprised by space alien zombies. The events have to be big. Like New York and California State Legislatures deciding to secede and the Feds saying no. Oregon sending its National Guard armored regiment over to Idaho to force Idaho's Electoral College Electors to certify a certain way and Idaho greeting them at the border with TOW missiles and A-10s. Or perhaps a very contested election that looks sketchy as hell even after a Supreme Court ruling. At any rate, we are talking some insanity that lights the fuse on this powder keg and takes us down a path that can't be stopped; open combat that eventually becomes Red County against Blue County against others.

A common mistake I think many people are making is the assumption that factions will be clean cut and obvious like in our 1861 Civil War. First of all, the lead up to that conflict was actually pretty messy. You had active terrorism for years prior on both sides known as Bloody Kansas. Political organizations existed in the North and South trying to push their will in each other's territory. The issue of Federal Supremacy had not yet been settled. At the time, any US Citizen was much more likely to feel loyal to his state than the United States as a whole. Ladies, love ya, but you were still pretty much property back then (no offense intended, just a statement of facts). It was pretty cut and dry that when a State left the Union, all its residents backed that play. Due to the way the military was organized at the time, each side ended up with a pretty much in-place military structure, ready to fight in the manner that 19th century warfare said they should.

Now there are many things that stay consistent across all time for human warfare, but a great many also change. It's not that guerrilla warfare didn't exist back then but it had fallen from vogue. Each side had a real army, so they didn't have to rely on guerrilla tactics. Not to mention the two teams were pretty much equals and there was not another major player on the field. What if Utah had taken the opportunity to declare itself a new Mormon nation in 1861? Would anyone have been able to stop them? What if Texas had said, "Nah, we want no part of this. We are back to being a Republic of our own"?

Sometimes, a conflict is very much between just two sides, even if one side is made up as a coalition out of convenience or necessity, such as the Irish War of Independence. However, the loss of Federal authority here could mean two factions or ten vying for control, not to mention organized crime and other opportunists just taking advantage of the chaos. You may have no idea yourself what the hell is going on.

Realistically, in a lot of ways, it doesn't matter how we arrive at this place. If law and order has become a bad joke and armed people are showing up to either take your shit or make you swear loyalty to some asshole you don't like, the conclusion is the same. You can either throw down your guns and bend the knee or you can shoot them. Most of you don't seem like the knee bending type. If I'm wrong on that, I guess I will be living in the Arctic Circle with the Inuits after this—or in a gulag.

How will you know you are in Phase 3? Well, I think it will be pretty hard to miss. Don't pop the cork early like a fifteen year old boy touching his first boob, but you really don't want to be behind the power curve here. People behind the curve in Phase 2 will get robbed. People behind the curve in Phase 3 will get killed or worse, disarmed and subjugated. There is an old saying in military circles: "Decide to be aggressive enough, quickly enough."

Some good indicators of legit Phase 3 happenings include obvious ones like a Governor declaring secession from the Union. Another might be State or City sanctioned militias acting in defiance of Federal authority. One might even extrapolate that to say burning down Federal Courthouses and expelling Federal authorities (looking at you again, Portland). A more subtle tell would be that you are now being shot at by things that don't exist in the United States like RPGs or Chinese machine guns. You may start finding obviously non-US nationals among the enemy, either as combatants or advisors. That is a pretty good indicator that someone else has entered the fray and it changes the calculus significantly.

Isn't the US Military going to protect us from this? In a great many possible scenarios, the military is an absolute wild card. If there is no clear winner of an election, who exactly are they supposed to take orders from? If it looks like a palace coup just took place, aren't they obligated to be loyal to the expelled President? This is one of the other places the Magic Paper fails, because we have never seen such a scenario pushed to fruition. Consider also that most of the Officer caste, especially the high ranking ones, are Blue team. While the vast majority of the rank and file are Red team. It isn't hard to envision a scenario in which the standing DOD forces split in such a manner as to effectively neutralize one another. Even if they don't start killing each other on day one, that makes the military as we know it cease to exist.

This isn't without precedent either. Every coup d'état I can think of over the last fifty years has had at least parts of the military side with the usurpers. While it is easy to judge that through our perfect lens of history, it also isn't hard to see how they could think they are doing the right thing in the moment. Add to that a reality that a lot of civilians don't have to face: if you are in the military and you pick the losing team, whoever that may be, your odds of being executed for treason just skyrocketed. On top of that, the last twenty years has taught us that as a military power we aren't all that great at fighting insurgencies anyway. It's just not really a strong suit for us. Coupled with desertions and outright defections, things could get really weird, really fast.

Now let's add the icing on the cake. Even in top form, how many cities do you think the entire US military could occupy at once? Ten? Twenty? I assure you, there are not nearly enough troops to quell what looks like 20% of the population of the United States—not on our best day. I could be wrong here, and maybe a single episode of the 82nd Airborne handing out some hickory stick shampoos could snap this insurrection overnight, but as the days pass I doubt it more and more. Both sides of the equation are absolutely fanatical right now and that usually only ends in blood—lots of it.

Even if the military is functional, it is likely to be overwhelmed. That would be different if the bad guy team would just put on some Blue or Red coats and meet them on the field of battle. You could sell that shit on pay per view and it would be over in about 48 hours. Our current military is exceptional at destroying conventional military formations. This is also why no one except a complete fucking retard would choose to fight them that way. Whatever you might think about the opposition forces, they aren't stupid; at least not up at the command and control levels.

Even if you are far from the fight, a power vacuum is likely to exist. If Atlanta is number eleven on the list but enough forces only exist to handle the first ten metro areas, you are still on your own. Power abhors a vacuum. Something will rise up to fill the hole left by an absence of Federal authority, be it a warlord or a cartel. Like death and taxes, it is inevitable. It wouldn't take all that long for us to become Mexico. The only real difference is that we aren't disarmed peasants, so we have a chance of not letting that happen.

No matter how it shakes out, the Blue Team centers of power are clearly the larger cities. A look at a map of voting records by county shows exactly where those are and therefore what are the likely hot spots. Armed with that knowledge, what are you going to do about it? If we had any sense, we would just wall off those cities and let them eat each other, and we would be doing it right now in Phase 1 so that Phases 2 and 3 never have a chance to even evolve. However, it is highly unlikely we will be able to muster the political will to do so until it is far too late. Besides, if we did, we would be leaving a lot of good people to die. I don't think that's palatable for us as a collective even if it is the right thing to do tactically. The longer this conflict goes on, the more you will learn this truth. The tactically correct thing to do is often not the morally correct thing to do. May your luck and judgment keep you alive and able to live with yourself after.

About this time, you are going to need the militia to take over from LE. This will no longer be a situation that is suitable for badges and due process. To quote Alejandro from the movie *Sicario*, "You are not a wolf and this is a land of wolves now." Some of your LE will embrace the new rules but many will be unable to change their mindset at first. The key is to help them survive long enough to learn.

The first problem, as with the other phases, is going to be refugees. On this front, you ain't seen nothing yet. If it felt like a flood during Phase 2, Phase 3 will be a Biblical event. Part of this stems from mindset. This will sound insane to you if you live in a rural area, but a huge percentage of occupants in major cities have *never* been outside of the concrete jungle. I would venture to say the vast majority, still in this day and age, will die within ten miles of where they were born. They just don't leave that comfort zone and it will take something huge to get them moving. History has shown that a no-shit shooting war is huge enough. A lot will still stay, no doubt—look at the occupants of Beirut or Damascus—but enough will beat feet to make your life complex, as the invasion of Europe over the last ten years illustrates. Unlike Phase 2 refugees, this will be a herd of humanity, much of it on foot, looking for anywhere but where they came from.

How much of this you have to deal with is directly related to your proximity to a metropolis. If you are the first small town outside New York City, it's going to be a tsunami. If you are further away, there is a lot of bleed off before it gets to you but he numbers may still be staggering. These people will be desperate in a way none of the other waves compare to. This is not the group you want setting up shop at your elementary school playground.

You aren't going to like what you'll have to do. Pretty much everything in Phase 3 is merciless so start hardening your heart now. General Tecumseh Sherman said it best, "War is cruelty and you cannot refine it." That sums up perfectly the mindset difference between a bright-eyed idealistic young soldier and a combat hardened veteran.

At this point, you really cannot afford to be taking in refugees outside of some very valuable and very unique skill sets, which you should be screening for. Beware of con artists; if you start asking for doctors, pretty soon everyone with a few hours on

WebMD is going to be pretending to be a doctor. The assumed safety of being inside the wire will make already desperate people do nearly anything to have it. So part of your screening process should be bringing down your own resident expert to question the hell out of any potential diamonds in the rough. I would be looking for medical personnel, soldiers, cops, machinists and chemists here. Your own needs will vary but this is something to think about ahead of time. I will also strongly recommend a reading of *Lucifer's Hammer* by Larry Niven and Jerry Pournelle on this topic.

As for the rest of the refugees, you likely can't feed them and if you try, it will be a massive drain on resources. More practically, you can't have a bunch of randos, at least a percentage of which are criminals or enemy sympathizers, loose inside your wire. You also can't stop them past a certain numerical advantage. Think about animals being pushed by a wildfire. That is roughly what it becomes if the city and its hooligans are like fire burning towards them and you try to just stop them alone. This has worked in places like Hungary against the hordes of North African refugees, but that required a lot of infrastructure to be built and a standing army to enforce.

What about shooting them? That fails for both moral and practical reasons. One, I very seriously doubt most of you have the wholesale slaughter of unarmed people in you, at least early in the war. Two, it would waste all the ammunition you are going to need to fight with later. What are you going to do if you spend 10,000 rounds just keeping scared people at bay and then have jack shit left for the armed component of Blue Team that shows up a week after?

So you are going to have to move them. Once again, the best way I can think of isn't an original idea. It is lifted whole cloth from *One Second After* by John Matherson, also an excellent read for understanding both how refugee waves could move and some good pointers on how things can fall apart logistically. The idea of moving them is to do so in such a manner that you have complete control of the situation and can get the bulk of them out of your area. It doesn't really matter where they go, as long as it is away from you. In this way, your little town or village is going to now resemble a Vietnam era firebase. The days of static front lines on long fronts ended eons ago; you only own what you can protect for 360 degrees.

Principally, you want them to see your town as someplace they can't stay. Pushing them in another direction makes it not your problem. The easiest way, if such is available, is to set up a checkpoint and point them to an alternate route around you. This works best if you have a bypass road that is sufficiently far enough away from your assets that they won't want to try and come in another way. The next best method described by Matherson is for if you only have one road going through your town. Line it with chainlink fence to create a narrow funnel and push your refugees through by groups of fifty or so, whatever you can handle without high odds of a prison break. For cars, you don't necessarily want to permanently block the roads in and out of your town (you may need out eventually too) but throwing up some serpentines will at least force anyone on approach to slow down. I'm guessing we are a ways off from suicide bombers; that takes not only ideology but know how.

You may also want to put out some hopeful signs like, "Next Gas, 30 miles" or "FEMA camp, 50 miles." This sounds like a cruel hoax but it is the lesser of two evils. A damn lot of people are going to die of exposure and they will turn feral before that. Best to have it happen not on top of you. The environment is a weapon too, so use it when you can.

Depending on your geography, you may not even be able to really push people down the road. If you are quite obviously the last stop before say, the Mojave Desert, anyone that shows up is staying. It might be a mile past where you forced them but that buffer isn't static. Also some of you could actually feed half the world, if not on milk and butter, at least on bread. Enid, Oklahoma has a population of 40,000 but boasts the third largest grain storage capacity in the world. They can afford to be a bit less of a dick. In those types of scenarios, you may want to make another plan of building a real refugee camp as opposed to a hobo camp, but still outside of your perimeter.

The difference will be this one much more resembles a prison. It needs to have wire and guards and a policy of 'if you go in, you stay in.' These refugees may also be needed as farm workers and harvesters later, which you should be upfront about. When things get rough, if you want to eat, you work. This sounds a lot like slave labor and is 100% contrary to the American way, I know, but your options are pretty limited here. You can't let a city of hostiles just spring up organically in your backyard anymore than you can divert labor to feed 10,000 hungry mouths in a makeshift prison. Nothing about this is good but you have to do the best you can.

At this same time, you need to have a serious chat with your merchants. Back in Phase 2, it would pay you great dividends to encourage them to keep about half of their supplies on hand to be sold to locals only. Especially with fuel, as that is going to be one of the greatest needs there is going forward. That could be as simple as limiting days open, raising the price for everyone not a local, whatever. It runs contrary to a merchant's instincts to not sell everything on hand but you have to try, especially as resupply gets less and less likely during Phase 2. Now in Phase 3, you need to consider not letting them sell critical supplies at all. Oof! That sounds exactly like what we are trying to prevent, asshole! I know, I know, but once again, realism trumps idealism. No one that grew up in a capitalist system is going to like hearing this, but gasoline and diesel are going to be critical war stocks and you can't let some doofus keep using them to heat his pool or smoke the tires or whatever just because he has a Visa card. Same goes for building supplies, tires, animal feed, anything that isn't made right in the area. Now think about this. It's highly discouraged to just take things at gunpoint. Even Mao would avoid that when he could. It is much better to have pre-arranged this or if you didn't, to make a deal via logic and barter. Don't take someone's livelihood and expect not to make an enemy. Maybe they are pliable to being the new Bulk Fuels Officer, under an overall Logistics Manager, with all the 22LR and free firewood that entails? Rule #1 of warfare in your backyard should be not to make an enemy when you can possibly avoid it.

Your general defensive posture by this point should look like something out of Mad Max world. If you can possibly do so before things get sparky, breastworks around the entire area you want to defend would be great. That is feasible in the smallest of towns but not so much around bigger ones. Hard point bunkers, easily constructed from dirt or concrete, will help you there. Hopefully if you live in such a place, the outer area of defense is some type of building material that stops bullets. That's not going to be the case every time but if it isn't, you can harden them in the manner I laid out in *Concrete Jungle* for urban areas. Around now, you should also be trying to bring people inward that live outside of what you can protect. Even my small town has houses that run for miles intermittently all the way down the valley. It would be nearly impossible to protect all of them. Staying out there alone, if things turn really ugly, is to be a sitting duck.

We will discuss a few specific skills you need to practice in a few chapters, but for now we are going to avoid any "you should do this" action. This is me once again bending to my legal team. Suffice to say that sometimes the best defense is a good offense and sometimes disrupting an attack far away from you is the best move—in Minecraft.

We do still need to talk about one thing that is critical here. Remember when I told you about Russia always losing the first 300 miles of territory and then smacking the invaders in the pee-pee once their supply lines are stretched? Your preferred defense should go the same way. We are going to simplify the shit out of the military term "Defense in Depth."

Wait, why can't we just reenact the Alamo at the house like they do on TV? You just said it yourself: they lost at the Alamo and nobody survived. I'm a native Texan, so don't @ me. They're heroes and all that, but dying in place is rarely the best move unless you absolutely have to buy time for someone else. You need to be flexible and understand that the numbers can be so lopsided that defending one particular location is absolutely impossible. Even if we dropped in the entire Ranger Regiment for you, the numbers can be so big on the other side that even they would be overwhelmed by an enemy armed with only slingshots. Defense in Depth is a way to cede ground while making your opponent pay for every single inch of it.

The easiest way I can think of to explain how this is done is to give you a highly fictional hypothetical which you can also follow along with on a real-world map. We do this all the time in military training, so don't read anything into the specific scenario, but I would encourage you to open up a map of the area on your computer and switch it to satellite view.

Let's say I live in Idaho City, Idaho, a tiny little place of like 400 people, and through training magic I have managed to turn all 400 into my little army (just to simplify the numbers). We are opposed by Boise, 35 miles away, who has amassed an invasion force of 50,000 to come and take our Ramen noodles. If we let that 50,000 hit us square on, our defense doesn't have a chance. Jesus could've dug those fighting positions personally and we are still going to get overrun. But those 35 miles give us a lot of breathing space due to some unique characteristics of the terrain. There is only one good road to Idaho City and only one secondary road that is worth mentioning. The big road is Highway 21, a two lane highway with a river on one side and steep cliffs on the other for most of its length. There is one primary bridge over the reservoir that is 200-ish yards long. That bridge is the first line of defense and it is a doozy.

The bridge can easily be protected by just a couple of dudes with scoped rifles on the hillsides between 600 and 900 yards away. If dug in, they would be hard to dislodge without artillery, especially if one of them is packing something for reliable vehicle interdiction like a 338 Lapua. That narrow little bastard of a bridge turns into a death trap. The opening salvo is to knock out the first vehicles in a convoy at about the mid way or ¾ point. Any closer and you may get some unfriendlies loose on your side of the river. If you smack them on the beginning of the bridge, it is easier for them to clear and try again. You've put them in a difficult spot of needing to clear wreckage in a killing ground to be able to move forward or abandon their own if they move back—not fun.

Now eventually, the enemy will figure out that they can dislodge you by foot moving down a mile or so to where the stream is crossable and flanking that position. This is still an uphill fight or a 1600 yard shot, both of which suck for them, but a dedicated enough force makes that happen. Now what?

Simple. We fall back down the ridgeline to the next channelized spot where we have already pre-dug fighting positions in the weeks ahead of this. By design, we have moved just far enough that the fortified spots we left can't reach us. So we have offered nothing of gain to the enemy and they have to come dig us out again. Our logging team has already created an absolute mess over the road with a couple of chainsaws or a rockslide, also easy to start in this place. Enemy forces consolidate after they clear the bridge and run right into another well prepared defensive situation. Let's say they eventually figure out how to circumvent it and clear. Fine. There are nine choke points on the route to Idaho City without stretching what is possible. That is a lot of time and a lot of blood to wade through, but let's say they are so dedicated they make it.

Either exhausted from relentless pressure or having been forced to stop and rest (buying us time and distance again), they arrive. Now they have to throw themselves at a *very* well fortified town and they won't find what they are looking for. As soon as forces started massing back at the bridge and it looked like we couldn't win, the rear echelon of women and children packed everything of value onto trucks and left as a convoy for the next town, Lowman, hours ago. Idaho City fights from its dug in positions until it looks like they will be overwhelmed, then collapses its defense and conducts an orderly withdrawal. Preferably they light anything they had to leave on fire as they shut the door. Half a mile outside of Idaho City is another choke point, which we pass through while waving at our allies from Lowman. Fresh troops are manning another series of defensive positions across the next 33 miles. All Boise has gained is a lot of frustration and useless territory, and they get to start all over if they have the stomach for it.

Sure, this is a simplification of the tactic. Couldn't Boise come over the mountains a different way on foot? Not with freshly minted soldiers, no chance. Plus, you'd be lucky to find 200 people in the Valley that could find Idaho City through the mountains without GPS. The force capable of being brought to bear would likely not be big enough to overwhelm a defended town. Could they go around? Half the state, maybe. Anything closer supposes they go through Horseshoe Bend or Garden Valley, which in this scenario are likely just as well defended.

With a little thought, this can apply everywhere. My place has unique terrain, one of the reasons I chose to live there, but even on the plains you could make this work. It might just be technicals (rifles on Toyota pickups) dug into tank style fighting positions, but it would work. Some places just digging up the road with an excavator could buy you all kinds of time.

There are absolutely situations where my scenario falls apart. It doesn't work for shit if the bad guys have armor or mortars and we don't also have Javelins and counter battery indirect. Even then, the principle is the same and my money is still on facing mostly irregulars. If for some reason the 3rd Armored Division shows up, you are probably fighting the wrong guys.

This is one tactic I am really giving a lot of ink to because it applies to all of you. If you are butted up to a Blue megacity, odds are you won't have the forces to stop them then and there, but you can slow them down. If you are the second, third or tenth city down the line, you need the same thing. If that group of 50,000 can drive to your front door unimpeded they are going to stomp your ass. This is about using time, distance and allies to bleed that wave off.

It makes sense to start coordinating with the towns to your left and right as well. Lowman needs Idaho City to mount that initial defense. It may even want to throw some troops in the mix as a measure of goodwill. Lowman better not treat Idaho City like refugees when they show up and not just for moral reasons. You don't want to have to fight some dudes that just got battle hardened over a period of weeks when they could be your allies. This is where the Red Counties had better start adopting a "Join or Die" mentality. Alone, any one of us is easily overwhelmed.

Together, the Blue team doesn't have a fucking chance if they turn this into a shooting match.

If Phase 3 goes this far, is going to be an absolute shit show. Just like in 1861, it is easy to turn off before the shooting starts. Even with secession, a political solution could have brought the Confederate states back into the fold right up until the attack on Fort Sumter. Historically, once the killing starts, it usually runs its course. I pray we don't find ourselves in that position but I also believe in keeping my powder dry and edges whet.

8   Combat Outpost Wheaties

One additional problem you have deserves some special attention. How will you protect farms and ranches that are by nature not going to be near your center of gravity for other defense? Them dudes have all the food, which is going to be an incredibly valuable resource as this situation develops. However, securing them presents its own challenges. First, they are generally out there, isolated, and they have to remain so to be able to take care of the crops, herd the emu or whatever. This isn't a medieval siege where you can just stack up some bags of corn and let the cows wander the town square until the bad guys leave. Our farmers and ranchers feed the entire world and the logistics of even being able to feed us say you can't cede all the growing land. Second, farmers and ranchers are by nature very hardheaded (looking at you, Braxton McCoy). Genetically, these are the descendants of the people that tamed the frontier. These are families that went beyond the limit of where the US Army could protect them because the land to do their business on was free. Even though they died, often in horrible ways, by the bushel full in Indian attacks, they stayed. These people usually can't be burned out, frozen out or scared off, so getting them to change their ways because some xi/xer twats from the city might come kill them is going to be an uphill battle. Even in the modern world, Boer farmers are murdered in South Africa at an alarming rate and yet they stay.

That said, the best course of action is going to probably be the Combat Outpost. This has its own limitations but can at least help the situation. A Combat Outpost is basically going to be a fortified little compound designed to keep the farmer alive long enough for reinforcements to be scrambled together in case of an attack. This would be made easier if you could consolidate farms, like having three to four families move in together to increase available manpower and cut down on the labor needed to secure them; but see above, notorious hardheadedness. The other glaring problem is that most farm and ranch houses were built with the goal of a good view or weather protection, not as a fortress against roving bandits. A house built in the lee of two hills is great for blocking blowing snow or strong winds, but is very easy to sneak up on and shoot down into. You have to work with what you've got.

Ideally, pick the most defensible house in terms of terrain to start with. Then a very not new idea is to toss up some defensive walls around said house, complete with a large inner courtyard. This is extremely common the world over. The ideal walls would be very tall and made out of mud or adobe, much like an Afghan qalat. While extremely labor intensive to create, those Afghan models are stunning. They are notoriously hard to breach even with military explosives and have been documented stopping bullets up to and including 25mm. Quite a feat considering 25mm makes 50 BMG look like a pop gun. The next best choice would be a T-wall or Bremer wall, the very tall concrete "jersey barriers" we commonly used in Iraq and Afghanistan to protect our own houses. With some ramparts on the top, this is pretty hard to beat, but I would say it is prohibitively expensive and therefore unrealistic as a goal. Therefore, at a minimum, you want to run with the qalat principle but probably just with dirt. Three feet high should offer some pretty decent protection from ground fire and give you a solid defensive position from which to fight back. I don't think I should need to say this is only going to help if you have someone on watch to detect an attack coming.

Educating the local farmers and ranchers about the principles of standing watch is going to be key. You can incorporate some technology to help here. The battery and solar power needed to run just a small security system is pretty minimal. With well-placed cameras over an open area, one person at a watch desk can cover a lot of territory. Cameras that can see in the dark are much cheaper than goggles that can see in the dark, and after dark is your primary threat. This can also be enhanced with some well thought out security lights. The motion sensor on a modern security light is a thing of wonder. Even the cheap ones are amazing. Unlike their intended use, I'm not talking about slapping them up right on the house or the corners of the qalat. Detecting a threat that close is not likely to help you much; you will be dead before you can mount a defense. The walls and fighting positions do nothing for you if the enemy is already inside them before you notice. I'm talking about stringing those motion lights out *way* outside of the house, 150 yards or more. If you have night vision cameras or are running goggles, you should replace the bulbs with IR bulbs. This gives you a long range visual alarm that your enemy can't detect unless they are also wearing goggles; very unlikely in the early stages, at least.

You can also go old school here for a significantly reduced price. Tin cans with pebbles in them on knee high fishing line is a classic. You can also buy twelve gauge blank shell trip wire alarms on Amazon, which are amazing. Just using your brain a little bit can deter most infiltration. Let us not forget geese and dogs as intrusion detectors.

Plan early on using a part of your overall force as either qalat protection or as herd protection. My prediction is that food is going to be a huge problem if this sparks off in earnest. Hungry people will also do desperate things. Even with just the COVID nonsense back in May, I had ranchers asking me about protecting their livestock. It's a big burn on manpower but allocating forces to this vital supply is going to be worth it. Having a cheeseburger in the winter of 2022 trumps a lot of other infrastructure, and that may include power stations and water treatment facilities (situation dependent). Don't underestimate the need here when you start thinking about priorities. Also don't forget that some crops are susceptible to fire when they are ready to harvest and it isn't out of the question they'll be targeted. Even if both sides are hungry, some 85 IQ warlord might decide destroying them is the tactical move. Once a war gets rolling, humans historically stop thinking about 2nd and 3rd order effects.

9   The Very Bad M-Word

We briefed over how and why to build a militia, infantry platoon and hatchet force earlier, but some further thought leads me to believe we need to extrapolate a little bit on exactly how to organize one and why. Now again, "militia" has taken on a very bad connotation over the last forty years. Just tonight, some retards alleging to be a Michigan Militia got caught hatching some Rube Goldberg-esque plan to kidnap the Governor, which doesn't make the word look any better.

We have to do this because the situation is different. In *Concrete Jungle*, I told you to stay away from large formations. This is 100% true, given the situation you would face in the city. If the war breaks out, you should be leaving the Blue strongholds if possible. This can reasonably be accomplished by one man alone if absolutely necessary. I could have very possibly walked across Baghdad in 2006 by myself and made it. I wouldn't want to try, and absolutely would not be assured of success, but the possibility existed. If this current set of shenanigans turns into a true Civil War, then that calculus changes. I can't fight the population loyal to Blue Team alone and neither can you. Nor can I do it with just my old twelve man team. We are going to need some serious numbers to counter whatever weight they can bring to bear. This remains to be seen after the first bullet flies but it looks large enough right now to at least take it seriously.

Is forming a militia illegal? Not even a little bit. Let's turn to the US legal definition of the militia as outlined in 10 U.S. Code 246: Militia: composition and classes:

" (a) The militia of the United States consists of all able-bodied males at least 17 years of age and, except as provided in section 313 of title 32, under 45 years of age who are, or who have made a declaration of intention to become, citizens of the United States and of female citizens of the United States who are members of the National Guard.

(b) The classes of the militia are –

(1) the organized militia, which consists of the National Guard and the Naval Militia; and

(2) the unorganized militia, which consists of the members of the militia who are not members of the National Guard or the Naval Militia."

Cool? Also let me reiterate this one more time: anyone that advocates for building bombs, illegal SBRs, off-the-books suppressors, unregistered machine guns *or kidnapping or murdering the goddamn Governor at his or her Summer residence* is either a Fed, an Informant or a nutjob and should be expelled immediately without the possibility of return.

"But wait dude, isn't all that gun shit an infringement?" Personally, I think you should be able to buy belt feds and RPGs at the local 7/11 while wearing a balaclava and not having an ID, but we have bigger problems right now and this isn't the time for that fight. We can work on fixing that as soon as we ensure Commies don't win and purge us all under the new soy boy Khmer Rouge.

Okay, on to organization. The best idea here is to not reinvent the wheel. The US DOD has spent the last 100 years conducting countless taxpayer funded Rand Corp studies to figure out how to make an infantry unit. Let's just copy and paste, giving it some tweaks where necessary—simple is good. First, who is going to run this goat rodeo? You can get away with some pretty loose leadership in a small unit or team. With bigger ones, you have to have a clearly defined chain of command or the whole thing falls apart. However, that doesn't mean you are going to have USMC level discipline and order—keep dreaming. A common mistake I often see with documentaries and news coverage of modern militias is exactly this. They have like a Saturday afternoon together and they spend it with Bob the Warlord inspecting the troops' guns for rust and all kinds of silly shit. Don't start thinking you are Big Sarge on Parris Island or your militia is going to quit.

A natural kind of hierarchy exists among military veterans, which hopefully you are lucky enough to have a few of in this building process. For the task at hand, it would go something like this:

1) SOF or Infantry guys
2) Other combat arms guys (tankers, Cavalry Scouts, Artillery)

3) Other jobs that carried a gun (MPs, Blackhawk Crew Chief, Gunners Mates)
4) Others, at least from a ground combat influenced service
5) Air Force veterans (eat me, BKactual).

Now this is no disrespect to anyone or any service, it's just how it works for the job we need. If we were making an airwing, I'd be the guy washing the windshield (if I'm even qualified to wash the windshield; that might require some special sauce I don't even know about). Not the point.

Along with jobs, you may have some wild or retired rank disparities that offset the above. If I am trying to pick the dude in charge, do I pick the E-3 Private Infantryman from the National Guard (1986-1989) or the recently retired Command Master Chief EOD guy? Despite the above matrix, I'm going Master Chief. How about if I have a full Colonel but he was a pilot? Probably not going to let him run my ground combat formation, but he would likely make a better regional commander than I would, flyboy status or not. This is mostly going to sort itself out, if you let it. Don't get all wrapped around the axle about who did what and remember to use the material you have on hand.

With the leader sorted out, now how do you organize? The first bit is your actual infantry unit and after that we will cover the supporting bits. Shouldn't every available swinging Richard be in your infantry, if things are so dire? Kind of. You can't push people into a role they are physically incapable of doing. While we aren't exactly holding 82nd Airborne levels of physical standards here, you are still going to find a number of people that just cannot possibly do even the baby step things you need an infantry to be capable of doing. You can still find a job for them, it just isn't on the shield wall on the lead edge of battle.

The structure of any infantry formation should be copied from DOD doctrine for simplicity. We are going to use some terms here that could be substituted but for ease, just incorporate them into your lexicon.

Squad is the basis for most of what we will be talking about later in tactics, so use that as your primary building block. A squad is thirteen men in a USMC infantry formation and nine in a US Army infantry formation, because the Army is dumb. They wanted a squad to fit inside a Bradley or some such nonsense. We are going to use the USMC narrative because it fits better. That thirteen man unit is made of three, four man fire teams (another block) and a squad leader. After that, the entire structure of a military is built on the principle of threes: three squads make a platoon, three platoons make a company, three companies make a battalion, three battalions make a regiment, three regiments make a division, blah blah blah... At least if we ignore some of what you don't need, like weapons companies, HQ elements and a bunch of other nonsense that would just confuse the issue at the moment, the odds of you creating something larger than a platoon to start with are slim and certainly nothing bigger than a company. By the time you have a bigger unit, the odds are certain that a veteran leader will be present to further help with organization.

Your squads and fire teams can be as big or as small as you need them to be. I know of one unit under construction that at the current time is fielding two man fire teams for the sake of simplicity. Two men in Phase 1, our current status, is enough to knock off problems. It also allows you to spread limited numbers around pretty well. Work with what you have and make it fit your needs. If you can field two such six man squads right now, great. If you only have one dude that really knows what he is doing, maybe you simply have one twelve man squad. Don't get too wrapped up in details right now, a start to organization is enough.

Each squad should have an assigned squad leader, which in this case is the dude who most knows his shit. If you have enough troops for multiple squads, there should also be (for lack of a better term) a Platoon Commander. This is just to make things easier on structure, and I would stop short of assigning ranks and nonsense like that. First off, slapping co-opted ranks on a militia is cringe as fuck, and second, it's rather pointless. You make yourself a Lieutenant but the guy down the road made himself a Captain. Driven by ego, you go home and make yourself a Colonel. Next thing you know, we are all Generals like in African wars with seven stars on the collar plus badges and stripes. It's silly.

The only real reason to even have this base leadership stuff is for simplicity of orders and to avoid having 25 people trying to talk at once. You will have to elect your own leadership; a tradition as old as actual combat. The Boers, when fighting the British, were prime examples of quite literally electing Captains on the fly. The Ranger Companies of the old frontier wars were another. At the end of the day, irregulars will only be led by charisma and personality.

Thinking you will get real military style discipline and order is a fool's errand. That only works in well-established hierarchies and only then because it is backed up by the literal consequence of a death sentence. For example, the Romans had a special helmet for officers. If I had the magic helmet, it was given to me with the authority of the State and that magic helmet meant I could order anyone with a lesser helmet to do anything I said. That's very handy if say, we are being overrun by barbarians and your own officers are dead. I show up with my magic helmet and order youse guys to cross that river or charge up that hill, and you do it because we have built in this hierarchy that allows such decisive action. See the Roman invention of the word "decimation" for a clear understanding of how this would work. Even in the modern militaries of the world, disobeying an order is actually punishable by death, as is cowardice in the face of the enemy. You will never, ever achieve that standard of discipline with irregular or guerrilla forces outside of perhaps Mao or the Vietcong. So don't try to do it and use other incentives that you can actually back up. Peer pressure alone has made for some incredible actions by irregulars in the past.

Again, we only have the organization because of simplicity. A phone tree is a Christmas tree shaped chart with one person at the top. He calls two people below him who each have lines drawn to them. They each call three people, and so on to the bottom. It makes it easy to ensure everyone is reached without one person having to make fifteen phone calls. If we make a phone tree for the purpose of spreading info, do we make calls at random or does the Commander call the Squad leader, they each call the Fire Team leaders and they each call the Fire Team members? This also prevents you from having to play pick up basketball every time a job needs done. Eighteen people are needed on Main Street, plus six to secure the pass into town. Which is faster:

"Johnson, Scalise, Goldberg... fuck, I already assigned Goldberg. Uh, Johnson again... Uh, you guys go secure Applesauce Gate. Everyone else with me."

or

"Johnson, your squad covers the pass. Martin, Goldberg, Vedder, you have Main Street. Ford, Daines, Smith, you are in reserve."

Plus it gives you someone to hold accountable when things aren't done to standard. Again, take the Applesauce Pass scenario. You tell Johnson to secure it and show up three hours later to find four dudes with lawnchairs in the middle of the road and two gone. Is it easier to give everyone a talking to or tell Johnson he is a fucking idiot and to fix himself?

The infantry part should be made of at least semi able-bodied men for reasons that will really be evident later. What about your other warm bodies? Fortunately, you have other needs, and it is also important to use all the resources you have. If you start every militia meeting off with a five mile run and a cold river swim, you will be leaving a lot of valuable talent at home watching foosball. Do you have, perhaps, some old varmint shooters that are too fat to walk a mile? They're not what you need in your infantry, but you have just gained a sniper or designated marksman section. You will want an intelligence structure, what the military would call an S-2. Old people and especially old women can take care of this.

They already have all the skills they need. How about working out all the logistics of survival not related to shooting? That would be an S-4. Time is a precious resource; just unscrewing all the supply needs of what is coming is a full time job. If you try to do that, plus get ready for a shooting match, you're probably going to do both half-assed. A great S-4 would be someone like a store keeper or a data entry person. Unless you have a gaggle of medical professionals, it's probably best to keep them off the front lines. A little medical platoon can be formed to both teach med skills and provide support during training.

If you can possibly swing it, I would make a concession to regular military discipline and order. If at all possible, get some type of uniform. This is helpful for two reasons. First, it makes everyone feel like they are a part of something professional. Unit pride and looking the same do matter in things like this. Second, it makes it easier to identify friend from foe. Even if we are talking head to toe camo, the human brain starts to recognize patterns over time. You are much more likely to be able to spot your own, even in dense foliage or whatnot, if your brain has had time to imprint a pattern, no matter how well that pattern happens to blend in. A lot of lives have been saved by the US military giving its uniforms to partner forces. Shooting people that aren't dressed like you is a lot easier than trying to make a snap judgment deciding if that's Bill from down the street or not. It will pay off later.

That being said, don't dress like goobers. There is absolutely no need to be in head to toe camo complete with grease paint every time you do some training together. Also for fuck's sake, do not ever tuck your pants into your boots. That is a near instant method of separating LARPing chucklefucks from people that are useful.

I suggest that you keep it simple and take a page from SF teams: Carhartt pants of whatever color you choose and a camo BDU top. Several Special Forces teams across my career ran exactly this set up, in theater. Carhartts are not only durable but everyone you know probably already has some. Good enough for Afghanistan, good enough for you. Pick a BDU top that is cheap, readily available and generally works for your area. Mil surplus is going to be your friend here and it really doesn't matter if it is multicam, desert or even some European pattern. Vote on it, make sure supply is plentiful and make it so. Not only do you avoid looking like some extra from a bad action movie, but you can shed a skin at will. Want to go grab some beers after training? Drop the camo top and you look like a normal dude again. Leave the Squeal Team 9.5 $400 assault pants to the airsofters and make this easy on everyone.

What about higher echelons, regional commanders, that sort of thing? Look, I have normally shied away from anything bigger than about twelve because of necessity, but I am now telling you to kick those numbers up. However, going outside of your immediate area is fraught with a different kind of danger. It can be negotiated but you have to tread very carefully on this one. If you start making a big regional or national organization and someone affiliated with it does some retarded shit, the hammer of the State can come down on you in ways you don't want. Anti-gang laws, RICO statutes, anything built to work against organized crime can equally be aimed at you, even if you personally didn't do anything wrong. The DOJ owns the image (patch) trademarks and property of several 1% biker gangs that fucked around and found out. Would you like to be in Bob's Midwest Militia and wake up on April 19, 1995 to find out Timothy McVeigh was a Regional Commander of the same organization one state over? No, no you would not.

There are exceptions to this rule but still, do your homework. American Contingency is a recent startup that looks like a winner. It was founded by my friend Mike Glover of Fieldcraft Survival Inc. whom I have known for about fifteen years. Mike is nobody's fool, so I am positive he has both looked at the legal angles as well as the potential risks. It's worth checking out as a starting point.

Train as often as you can and on a variety of tasks. The ones I think are most important are coming up next.

10 Whiz Bang Tactical Ninjary

Now that you are organized, we need to move on to individual tactics. This is an extremely difficult thing to learn from a book but also so absolutely necessary that I had to include the two tactics I think are most important for you. Each will get their own chapter. You can sort of learn them from a book, and it's better than nothing, but just intellectual knowledge is in no way enough. If I don't have an expert on hand and all I have is the book, I still have to go out and practice in the real world. While a book and book knowledge is in no way a substitute for an expert teacher, it still beats the pants off of having jack and shit in your quiver of options.

Tactics also require some dedication on your part to be useful. The best way I can think of to explain this is to use a jujitsu metaphor, assuming you have at least a passing understanding of the art, which in the age of UFC streaming is highly likely. Comparisons are fraught with danger and sometimes serve to confuse the issue more, but hopefully this helps here.

Let's call each tactic the equivalent of a jujitsu submission. If I'm new and I go to class and learn a basic armbar, can I use it twenty minutes later? Not well; it may work against an equally unskilled opponent who doesn't know how it works either, but with my slow and sloppy execution it also has a high chance of failure against even an untrained rival. An armbar looks like three steps to the uninitiated. In the same way, tactics written on paper look deceptively simple to anyone that has never tried to use them. In reality, an armbar is about twenty steps, many of them things like subtle weight shifts, body placement and pressure, etc. All tactical maneuvers are also full of subtlety when done well. I'll put in as much as I can without turning this into a ninety page chapter that includes what color your underwear should be.

Knowing intellectually how to do an armbar and being able to do an armbar are two separate things. When I first learn to perform an armbar correctly, it is going to take a lot of thought. That means it will be slower than Christmas wading through molasses while on Quaaludes. It isn't really going to be useful to me until I have done it *perfectly* about a thousand times in practice. Tactics are the same way. You are going to have to spend the hours rehearsing them before you are remotely competent.

Jujitsu is also a great way of understanding how tactics flow. Every tactic has a counter tactic. If my opponent does X, I can do Y and that negates X. An ambush can be broken and an assault repelled, but the real question isn't if you know said tactic, it is how fast and skillfully you can execute it. It's about knowing when it is the right move and when you are falling for a feint. Even professional fights are often settled by what looks to the layman like a very basic submission; an armbar or a rear naked choke, for example. It isn't that both fighters don't know those basic moves and how to counter them, it is that one eventually outruns the other's ability to see it coming (processing speed) and to counter in time (athletic skill).

That isn't the end of the grappling comparison. Just knowing a tactic also doesn't mean it can't be used against you. Skill offset at execution is a thing. Your ability to both quickly command troops and have them listen to your orders is equivalent to seeing a submission coming. Just understanding what is happening won't help you if you can't move things to counter or have an instinctive defense to a submission attempt. That is roughly equal to having practiced a tactic so many times that you are employing it before your conscious mind even tells your body to move. In our case, a reaction to contact (gunfire) which militarily is known as an Immediate Action Drill. Submission is 95% of the way to finishing you (you failed to recognize a ground attack and the enemy is inside your perimeter). You can still counter and win if your troops are better trained (you are strong, athletic and know the escape). For a wrestler this means energy and perhaps pain, but for you in a tactical situation, it is likely to cost blood and casualties.

I hoped this comparison helped. I can't really see another way to break it down. While we are on the subject, what is more important, tactical knowledge or individual skill? It depends; both are equally important in the right situation. Tactics are what you use to keep from getting yourself in a bad situation. Excellent tactics work with even mediocre skill. Skills are what you use when your tactics fail so that you don't die. Trust me, eventually your tactics will fail. As a GWOT veteran, I have been on the receiving end of more ambushes than I have hosted and I'm still alive. Keep that in mind too.

Alright, that was a lot of introduction to this chapter's lesson. The most basic of all infantry maneuvers, one that is so common it is practiced by everyone from USMC cooks to the British SAS, is Fire and Maneuver. Fire and Maneuver is the common link to any modern military set of tactics. Erwin Rommel is often credited with its invention during WW1. It was used by both sides of the conflict in WW2, if perhaps better than most by the German Army. Since then it has been perfected by Western armies and is among the first things a soldier will learn after how to tie his boots.

I was actually shocked to learn that most police don't know this day one soldier task. After the BLM massacre of police officers in Dallas back in 2016, I actually added this to the training schedule whenever I taught LE classes. Even a few hours of practicing Fire and Maneuver would have ended that attack very quickly. This just happens to be something that police are not taught, and it should be telling that a junior woodchuck Reservist carpenter with some half-assed basic Army training was able to kill five police officers and wound another nine.

To help you visualize this tactic, it would help to sit down at your kitchen table with some props. To start, place a salt and pepper shaker at one end of the table together. On the other end of the table, place another spice of a different color, like cumin. The odd color represents an objective, dug in enemy you need to assault. The salt and pepper represent two of you, for the moment. Broken down to its most basic level, Fire and Maneuver goes like this: Salt and Pepper both start by laying down (prone) or on a knee. Salt starts firing at Cumin on the far end of the table while Pepper gets up and sprints for three to five seconds. Pepper's objective here is to cover some ground, but only moving long enough for Cumin to be unable to get a good bead on him. This is aided by the fact that Salt is hammering Cumin's position with suppressing fire, hopefully keeping him behind cover and unable to get a clear shot. Pepper makes his move, drops to the prone position and starts shooting at Cumin. When Salt hears Pepper open up, he jumps up and runs forward for three to five seconds while reloading. Then he drops and starts shooting again. Pepper once again stands up and sprints, reloading while he goes, so on and so forth, until either they are so close they can shoot Cumin in the head regardless of his well built fortification or Cumin realizes he is screwed and runs away.

Seems pretty simple, right? In basic principle it is, and it absolutely works. Now let's complicate things a bit. Now I want two salt shakers (Team A) , two pepper shakers (Team B) and two of whatever you have that is red (Team C). Cumin is still the objective down at the far end, while Salt, Pepper and Cayenne represent the fireteams within a squad. Starting from the same position, now Salt and Pepper start shooting (base of fire) while Cayenne (both shakers) jump up and run. Ah ha! We have to have entire teams running now or we will never get there. Cayenne drops and engages while Pepper gets up and sprints. Meanwhile, Salt merely slows down its rate of fire so it doesn't run out of ammo before Pepper gets set. Pepper completes its movement and Salt gets up and sprints, and so on to the end of the table. Do you see how this can get complex?

To learn this with people, you clearly have to go out and do it. Before we get into how, I am going to go ahead and put this disclaimer in: I do not recommend you do this with live fire—*ever*. It is easy to get cocky thinking you got it dialed in when you don't. In the military, you would practice this all day for weeks with empty guns and blanks before they ever let you have a real bullet. Even in the infantry, it was not uncommon to do dozens of blank fire runs before one with live fire and people still die learning this. It is very easy to fuck up and run in front of your own guys and very easy to also not realize a friendly is fucking up by running in front of your muzzle. On top of which, it is very costly for ammo. How much 5.56 does it take to cover 100 yards of ground behind a wall of lead? More than you might think. Infantrymen burn up mountains of bullets staying proficient at this. At today's ammo prices that is unthinkable. Good substitutes for training are Airsoft guns or paintball guns, which provide enough sting to keep you on your toes. You don't even have to have that, just getting out and walking through it is going to reveal a lot of shortcomings.

To start, I usually use an open field with fake obstacles for cover: blue barrels or short plywood walls, whatever you have handy. While I start with empty guns, I do have the students do the empty gun magazine change so that they start to visualize how fast it needs to happen and how much more difficult it is to reload while sprinting. Start like we did with the salt and pepper shakers as individuals. Then when you have that down, move to two man or four man teams moving together.

Once you've got that down, try it in the woods, paying particular attention to how hard it is to move forward while not zigging or zagging into friendly fire. This is called 'staying in your lane.' You have about five feet on either side of you to maneuver in space before you risk getting shot in the back.

How nutty can this get? With combined arms included, it can get absolutely bananas. Imagine assaulting forward in this manner toward your own machine gun fire. It's firing perpendicularly (the flank) and it has to shift at the right moment or else it cuts you down too. Meanwhile a mortar barrage is dropping on the target, then rolling off the back to prevent enemy escape just at the right time as you go over the top of the defensive position, face shooting or bayonetting everyone that survived the onslaught—at night. This is a task we routinely give 18 year olds in the military, in a training environment supervised by maybe one or two Sergeants per element. An infantry combined arms assault is a horror to behold, so I strongly suggest you learn how to use this magic.

Fire and Maneuver is the the basic building block for everything else. If we run into a bigger force than us and we need to get away, the military term is "Break Contact," and it is exactly Fire and Maneuver in reverse. Our Salt and Pepper shakers start out close to the Cumin. One lays down a base of fire while the other runs *away* for three to five seconds. We do that until we are out of range and can just haul ass. If we're walking through the woods and we take contact from our right or left, it's an ambush. If it's a far ambush, as in a little distance away, we turn into the ambush and execute an Immediate Action Drill, which is Fire and Maneuver without talking about it. By doctrine, to respond to a near ambush, you just immediately assault through—or die. You wanted a flanking maneuver? Cool. Half our force lays down suppressing fire while the other half runs in a big circle to catch the enemy on its side (flank). They then sneak up until they the enemy spots them and then... Fire and Maneuver. Learn it, know it, love it.

I will close with this. Fire and Maneuver is so base a tactic that it is actually written into the mission statement of the USMC Rifle Squad. "The mission of the Marine Corps Rifle Squad is to locate, close with and destroy the enemy by Fire and Maneuver or repel the enemy assault by fire and close combat." Both sides of the coin, which should tell you how much you need to know it.

11   Regulators, Mount Up

The second important military tactic you need to understand is how to patrol. For our purposes, a patrol is a movement from point A to point B with some type of purpose. While military doctrine has about fifty different types, we are going to focus on just three, with one as a subset of the other. We will be discussing this as foot mobile as well as mounted (truck, horse, whatever) kind of interchangeably because your own solutions will involve a mixture of both while the fuel lasts. The principles are the same for both with some minor tweaks. Don't think, like the services did, that you only need one or the other. Prior to the GWOT, we mostly trained like we were going back to 'Nam: helicopter inserts followed by Sneaky Pete patrolling in dense foliage. Only to suddenly be surprised by a very mechanized war in two very different environments. That being said, I assure you that any veteran of either theater did some long foot work at one point or another, but 99% of us had to learn the bits about using trucks from scratch after the war had started.

For simplicity, I will also mostly talk about a small patrol of six to eight troops. Any type of patrol can be scaled up in size or scaled down for the most part, especially early in the conflict. The tactical situation of something like Phase 1 or 2 is significantly different than what you will face in Phase 3. While you might get away with a two man truck patrol early on, by Phase 3 that would be a minimum of two trucks carrying three men each.

The three types of patrols you need to learn to cover 99% of your bases are Recon, Security and Show of Force. Show of Force and Security are nearly identical, so we will combine those two with the minor differences highlighted as we go.

A Show of Force patrol is roughly the same thing as a uniformed cop walking his beat or driving around town at night; just showing a presence. Cops still stumble into a surprising amount of crime that way, though the real value is the crime they deter. Nobody is going to take the 30 minutes to try and steal an ATM if statistically a cop car drives by every 31. The neighborhood watch in day glow yellow shirts I talked about back in Phase 1 is a Show of Force patrol. It's you flexing nuts because the tactical situation says you can get away with it, and using the fact that you aggressively patrol your sector to deter incursions.

With a Show of Force patrol in a mounted setting, you might be driving with the headlights on, jackrabbit spotlights out the window, not even trying to hide what you are doing. Checking the infiltration routes, as we talked about earlier, and just generally being out there. You still want to vary routes and times to throw people off via unpredictability; it's more of a deterrent if no one knows exactly when. The foot mobile equivalent would be daylight patrols walking the area immediately outside your wire or patrols that take the obvious roads and trails. Right about now, you might be thinking this is a good way to get ambushed or blown up, which is absolutely true. Depending on the local security situation, we did do things exactly like this in Iraq. Like anything on the tactics side, it is a judgment call. Once things escalate to the point that getting your ass shot off for having the headlights on is a real possibility, it's time to shift gears to the Security Patrol.

The difference is that the Security Patrol is just a bit sneakier and stronger in numbers. Think like twenty to thirty goons; enough so that even if a small force hits first, hitting you at all is assured destruction. For mounted, you might be moving with headlights off but you aren't shy about getting out the lights at chokepoints to look for footprints or clothing on wire. If on foot, you aren't banging pots and pans together, but moving 25 people isn't exactly subtle. You will be moving a little slower to avoid walking into an ambush, but not as slow and quiet as a Recon patrol. A Security Patrol is still out there looking to cause some trouble, it is just subtle enough to hopefully set the terms of the start of the fight.

A Reconnaissance Patrol is a purposeful patrol to either see what is going on in a particular area or get some eyes on a very specific place for intelligence reasons. It could be a walk around in circles down by the highway to see if you can find evidence of a large enemy movement, or it could be a deliberate push into a Blue area to see if, for example, they have a UN food resupply at a warehouse. Regardless, the point of a Recon patrol isn't to get in a gunfight. The point is to avoid one if you possibly can, because the intelligence value of whatever you are looking for is more important than body bagging some purse-snatcher level bad guys. This is why a Recon Patrol will be very small, usually four to six men. It's large enough to do all the tasks that need doing but small enough to hopefully avoid detection.

Like I said earlier, all patrols are basically organized the same. I can even turn you to a very good resource besides me for how to organize one. Get a pre-1997 or so Boy Scout manual and read the patrol section. Replace all the sectors of observation with sectors of fire and bam! You have a military patrol. This isn't by accident; up until recently in its history, the Boy Scouts were acknowledged to be a paramilitary organization. Everything they taught could easily be converted to a military operation. This is also why Eagle Scouts received an instant promotion to E-3 in every US military service when they completed basic training.

For a foot patrol, the Point Man is up front. He doesn't get any other jobs, including navigation, because his one job is so important. He has his eyes peeled to make sure you don't stumble into an enemy force unexpected, step on a mine or hit a trip wire. It takes all the brain power one man can muster in a hostile place just to do that.

Behind him is the Compass Man. His primary job is to know where you are, where you are going and to steer the Point Man with his hands via arm signals from five meters behind him. This is the only person on the patrol that walks most of the way glued to his compass. He is reliant on the other patrol members not to let him get shot, as his awareness is generally used up on navigating.

Next is the Team Leader. He is centrally located for command and control purposes. Being right in the middle makes it easy for him to call halts or breaks and run the show when the shooting starts. His close proximity also allows him to easily communicate with the Compass Man and Point Man.

Fourth in military patrols is the Radio Man. He's located next to the TL (Team Leader) so he can call HQ, get air support, whatever. You don't have any of that, nor likely a gaggle of radios, so this is kind of irrelevant. I would make this my alternate Pace Man; he's the guy who specifically counts steps so you know how far you have gone.

Fifth is the Slack Man, usually put in this relatively safe spot either because he is the new guy or because he is the one carrying some unusually heavy load. Like let's say you have something you had to recover that can't be broken down for cross loading, like an aircraft black box. The poor bastard that has to hump it goes here, since he is most likely to be paying attention to his aching shoulders and not the woods around him.

Last is rear security, usually the Assistant Team Leader (ATL). This is a place for the second most senior and with-it dude on a team, for obvious reasons. He has two jobs: number one, to make sure you aren't snuck up on from behind and number two, as best he can, to counter track your patrol route. He picks up loose strings, wipes footprints when you cross a road and corrects bent vegetation while also paying attention to the direction and movement of the patrol. You want somebody with their shit together here.

What about the organization of a larger patrol, like the Security patrol we mentioned earlier? Well the first three positions stay the same, with the overall Commander right behind the Patrol Leader, then a mess of goons and the last spot is taken by whoever you designate as the Assistant Patrol Leader. It can be a bit more complex than that.

For a Recon Patrol, you are mostly going to walk in a file or single line, which is great for minimizing footprints and other signatures but sucks for bringing all your firepower to bear. Actually, it brings all the firepower of four to six dudes fast because you don't have much. It minimizes that ability when you get to larger numbers. Think of a line 25 people long, five meters apart (the distance you want so that one grenade or burst of automatic fire doesn't kill two of you), as a gun fight starts all the way up at the Point Man. Before the last guy in line even has a chance of a clear shot, he has to run 125 meters to the front. So a larger patrol can have a lot of variations of shape. Which briefs well, and all the manuals will tell you when to use them, but in the real world, you are probably going to be in two lines parallel to each other at best. Hell, I've seen terrain force Infantry Officers that swore, *swore,* they would never use a column into a single file line 36 Grunts long! You start getting fancy with the shape of the patrol and people will get lost, stumble into each other, all kinds of nonsense. So for amateur patrol hour, just stick to one or two lines. By the time that is no longer tactically a good idea, I'm sure you will have evolved.

It's reasonably straightforward how this translates to vehicles. The driver, regardless of which vehicle in the convoy he is in, just drives; one job and one job only. In the first truck beside the driver is the navigator. If you have space, right behind him in the back seat is the Team Leader or Patrol Leader. Military trucks make the security part easy: we have a turret built in with a machine gun. You are going to have to improvise with the classic Toyota Technical. First truck in line, at a minimum, gets a gunner either in the pickup bed or in a cut out sunroof. Everyone after that fills in and the last truck gets a rear facing gunner—easy peasy.

Then what? Well... patrol. Look, I could write an entire book on how to do this further because I've spent several thousand hours in the woods with grease paint and a giant ruck on. You are only really going to learn by doing. Same as Fire and Maneuver, this is a skill set you have to get out and practice. Take your Team or Militia on a tactical hike as often as you can. Learn to be quiet, by trial and error. Pick up a Ranger Handbook and use it to learn hand and arm signals. The fewer words spoken on a patrol, the less your chances of dying. Professionals can go days without a spoken word using just their hand movements to communicate. Use a paper map and get accustomed to always knowing where you are. While you are learning, take administrative breaks to do so. Drop security and talk it out so that everyone involved knows where you are. Pick up an Orienteering book and use it to learn terrain association. When your brain is really sharp at it, you don't even really need a compass anymore. Learn how spread out you can be depending on your local terrain. Learn how to keep the Compass Man closer to the Point Man at night, within touching distance, so he can keep the patrol on track.

This is important and it is going to take hours and hours of practice to get even decent at it. Start as soon as you can and do it as often as you can.

12   Redneck Cong Starter Pack

With the tactical stuff out of the way, we can now address the fact that you need some specialized stuff to make this happen. Remember when I said not to get out the Visa card? Well right after this chapter, it is time to get out the Visa card. I can see the glee in some of your eyes—try to keep it in your pants, gear queers. We gonna play dress up for your Carhartt Guerillas. Jokes aside, you do need some equipment. To my knowledge, the website *American Partisan* coined the term "Modern Minuteman Kit," and I can't think of a better one. Kit in this case is a term we borrowed from the British that means "all your personal war shit." If you say "kit" instead of "gear," everyone will know you are cool (pro tip—you are so welcome).

The advice for what to buy is plentiful out there on the interwebs and I'm not going to pretend to be the resident expert on every whiz bang, run faster, jump higher development in the Gucci gear market, mostly because I don't care. I didn't care when I was in and I don't care now. Give me some semi-decent stuff and I will get the job done. I'm not going to rebuild my kit I have been using for five years because the Version 2.0 Beta Test model saves half an ounce. I'm also loath to encourage you to spend several thousand dollars on this year's hottest Commando flavors when those precious coins could have gone somewhere more useful. I'm going to recommend the minimums but I'm also going to give you enough. Everything I put out as a need to have will have a very cheap option included.

The first question I get when people ask about kit is what plate carrier? A plate carrier is the slimmer version of modern body armor, essentially a nylon shell "carrier" to hold a set of ceramic bullet resistant plates. Disagreeing with many of my peers, I'm telling you that you don't need one. If you already bought one, fine, cool, no sweat, but I wouldn't make getting one a high priority. Opinions are like assholes, everybody has one—but you paid for my asshole opinion, so at least hear me out. Body armor worked well for us as soldiers because we were young, strong, conditioned to wearing it and mostly working in a dry heat. Would any of us have worn it if we were fighting in a Southeast Asian jungle? Probably not, because armor traps heat like nothing else. With ceramic plates front and rear, all wrapped in a thick nylon shell, it is basically an oven. We have shown that you can get away with that in the desert, but a blazing sun in a Louisiana swamp doesn't sound fun. Being conditioned to wearing it matters too. It takes a fairly serious amount of hours to adjust to be able to wear armor for long periods of time, and a bit of relearning how to climb, shoot, etc. We might have done some crazy feats of running or fighting in it, but we had the hours logged to know how. No matter how strong you are, that twenty pounds of armor will cost you some mobility. Given the parameters of the coming conflict, I would rather you be light and fast than slow and protected.

I also don't know that many people that took a direct strike from a bullet and lived because the armor stopped it. I know a lot of dudes; I used to ask this question when I was on instructor duty to my 300 or so students per year. The number is shockingly low considering the average number of tours per student at that time. It might've stopped some IED frag or other shrapnel but bullet strikes were low. You don't have to worry about much except bullets for the immediate part of the festivities. All that combined means to me that armor is not the best bang for your buck. If you insist, look at Hesco special threat plates or Angel Armor, and a quality carrier.

What do you need then? Pretty simple. Either a chest rig, a belt kit or both if you really want to have your bases covered. For a chest rig, I prefer the Mayflower/Velocity systems split front. The zipper bit allows it to stretch over winter clothing and the internal Velcro pocket system gives it flexibility. The inserts fit 7.62x51, 556 or AK mags and it has enough other real estate for my med kit and other little odds and ends. For a belt kit, you have two options. I still have an old school VTAC Brokos belt that I've been using for years. It is a little bigger than modern stuff but it is comfy. If you want the latest and greatest, the micro battle belts from companies such as Volund Gearworks are legit. Whatever belt kit you choose, make sure you buy the 308 size mag holders. 308 pouches hold 308 or 556. The same is not true in reverse. Some 308 pouches will also squeeze in an AK mag; a nice bonus if you have a gaggle of guns.

Whatever kit you get, resist the temptation to cover every square inch in pouches. The less nonsense you are carrying, the lighter and quieter you will be. My belief is that you should be carrying no more than four rifle magazines plus the one in your gun. Five total mags will get a lot of work done. We sometimes carried more in the jihad, but we also couldn't just melt into the mountains when things got protracted.

In addition to the mag pouches, you need two canteens. Carrying water isn't popular with cool guy kit these days, but that ignores that we've fought for the last twenty years with pallets of bottled water. If you didn't go overseas, I'm serious. In a move that would shock our Vietnam forefathers, we quite literally had pallet yards full of Avon bottles to pull from. It's basically a disposable canteen that fits in your pocket. You have no such luxury, so don't skip this step.

If you want to really skimp on money here, go get a Vietnam era H-harness and cartridge belt. The old stuff still works and works just fine. In fact, most every Special Operations qualifying school I know of *makes* you use the old stuff. You don't get to take Gucci kit to BUD/S, Amphibious Reconnaissance School or the Q course. You might get that stuff issued later, but when you are learning the ropes it is all last generation at best. If it is good enough for those environments, it is good enough for you. An H-Harness, belt, mag pouches and canteen/pouch set up should cost you about $50.

You need a good fixed blade knife, more so than even what I went over in *Concrete Jungle*. Do you know the difference between a fighting knife and a utility or combat knife? A fighting knife makes a shitty utility knife, but a utility knife will still stab the hell out of someone. Most of the time, your knife is going to be used for cutting rope, unjamming vegetation out of the prop of the boat, skinning a deer or some other utility task. Very rarely, if ever, is it going to be used to jab some asshat in the jugular. So pick the knife that does both jobs pretty well. Don't buy some huge Rambo knife; weight matters. Before you put a knife on your belt, weigh it and see how many equivalent rifle mags it could be. A blade five to seven inches long is plenty, and cheap options are good enough.

Not like gas station cheap, like original Ka-Bar cheap. If it was good enough to bring the Japanese Empire to its knees, it's good enough for you.

You will also need a backpack, aka a ruck. I like Eberlestock but something from the used sporting goods store is fine. Or a mil surplus ALICE, we are old friends too. Most of the time, you can even get away with a frameless model. Military packs are big because soldiers have to carry all kinds of heavy stuff like radios, radio batteries and rounds for the 60mm mortar, none of which you have to worry about. If you get a smaller bag, you will be less tempted to fill it with junk.

What goes in the bag? I recommend a poncho, mil surplus if you can find it. This is not just emergency shelter, it is to block the light if you are looking at a map at night. You will be doing so under a double layer of ponchos with a red lens flashlight. Speaking of, pack a couple of little red or green photon lights. Red and Green affect your night vision the least and are the least visible at distance. Pack a Gore-Tex jacket as a light warming layer. Include two more canteens, which fit rather neatly in the outside pockets of an ALICE pack, and a life straw or small Katadyn water filter. For other personal kit, pack a lensatic compass and maps of your immediate area, preferably laminated ahead of time. If not, put them in a secure, clear map pouch. Include a fair bit of grease paint. I'm a snob here, I always used the super Gucci liquid stuff they sell to bow hunters. The mil surplus stuff is fine too and is orders of magnitude cheaper. You'll want a couple of sets of mechanics' gloves in a non-fruity color, unless you also want to grease paint your hands. Pack some warm stuff, region dependent.

This is a shitty one, but no getting around it. I am generally not a fan of technology, but one piece is an absolute must if you possibly can. And it isn't cheap. Night vision aka see in the dark goggles. Nothing in the last 50 years has changed warfare as much as NVGs. And you absolutely cannot fight people that have them, if you don't, with the lights out. Even hadj knew this and started importing cheap Russian and Iranian devices as fast as they could. Because we were absolutely massacring them before they found a countermeasure. A set of goggles with a laser is more important than 20 extra guns or 50 pallets of ammo. If push actually comes to shove, this is just about the most important thing you can have on hand.

The best available option to most of us is a PVS-14, with a helmet, and a decent laser. Like a Steiner D-Bal or some equivalent. Which will set you back about $3000 for the goggles, $200 for the helmet and mount, and another $1200 for the laser. Which is well above what a lot of you could hope to spend.

Cheaper option? One does exist. And while it is nowhere near as good, it is enough to get you by. A Sionyx Aurora "night vision camera", which just happens to mount via aftermarket products to the same helmet. And if you absolutely have to cheap out on the laser, a Streamlight TLR-VIR II will set you back about $400. I have reviews up on this set up over on the YouTube, check it out. This set up is still over $1000, but I assure you, it will be the best money you ever spend.

On your feet, you need some season appropriate boots. You likely already have some, duh. If you find a set you really like, try to set aside the funds to buy three more sets. Shoes will be in short supply if this kicks off and we already saw weakened supply chains during COVID. If you can possibly have five years' worth of footwear on hand, do so. Making shoes locally is a lost art that some of us are going to sorely regret before this ends.

A personal rifle is a given and so important that it gets its own chapter.

Now I need to go on a little bit of a rant here but it's worth saying. After the last book, I got asked about all kinds of equipment like what tent or which JetBoil model, etc. which was initially very shocking to hear. Then I was perhaps a little bit angry that people assume this is a camping trip. But after some more thought, that is probably the only frame of reference most people would have.

So I'm not saying any of this to be a dick, I'm saying it so you understand the harsh reality. You aren't going to need any of that shit. You aren't even going to need a sleeping bag unless you live somewhere it gets frightfully cold. Even if you do end up using a sleeping bag, you aren't going to zip it up all cozy, you are going to drape it over the top of you. A sleeping bag can quickly become a body bag if you can't get out of it fast enough to fight. You aren't going to cook your food. Warm food has an aroma that carries for miles and hungry people will pick up on that. You are going to eat whatever you have cold and fast to minimize the signature before you stick it in a plastic bag and tape it shut. You will never once have a camp fire unless someone falls through the ice and it is decided to risk warming them up at the potential cost of everyone's life. There haven't been warming fires on the front lines since before WW1 due to the detection risk it poses. Cold camp will be the order of the day. Even that Gore-Tex jacket isn't to keep you comfy, it is to put on after you move all night through a rain storm so your chattering teeth don't give your position away on watch.

Gore-Tex is loud when you move and is an unacceptable risk. The poncho is not for a shelter unless it's so cold and rainy you'll die otherwise. Ground shelters are easily detected by the human eye, no matter how camo colored they are. A tent? Maybe if you are working in sub-zero temperatures.

The life of a soldier is one of suffering and discomfort. I wish we could make the people pushing for this conflict realize that before we all get more of a taste of it than we would like.

13   Cowboy the F*ck Up

A vastly underrated trait for the upcoming animated contest for freedom is mental toughness, including durability. I do get asked, on occasion, if I think it is an inherent ability or if it can be built. In my opinion, while it is a little bit of both, it absolutely can be improved just like anything else. Genetics might play some role in your ability to squat heavy or run fast but training is a factor as well.

This is also another example of rural types perhaps overestimating their own ability. I'm not trying to talk shit but I do want you to take a hard look inside. It is better to be insulted a little bit right now and have the capacity to fix it than to find out later your kung fu is actually weak sauce and you pay dearly for it. Does being from a certain area imbibe you with inherent toughness? Now that may have been true 120 years ago, but now not so much. Our luxurious lifestyle, particularly after WW2, has made us a soft and weak people. Let me go into story time mode to illustrate my point.

When I was a young USMC Infantryman, one of the first things my battalion had on the schedule was a winter mountain warfare package. Just by the name you can tell it was not going to be a fun time. And in the way that young Infantrymen deal with one another, the shit talking commenced from all the dudes from places like Michigan and Wisconsin. "I'm from the frozen North, this shit is old hat to me, but you gonna die Texas boy!" Which to 19 year old Clay, did sound like a real possibility. Fuck, I've never even seen the frozen North! I started prepping myself mentally. I made my roommates turn off the heater and we slept with the windows and doors open to our barracks room for a month prior to the event. That's not a huge sacrifice in North Carolina in December, but it was what we had. Flying out, I am not to proud to say I was perhaps a bit nervous that I would be able to perform in this new and scary environment. And you know what happened? Every one of those dudes folded like a cheap suitcase. Yes they were from Michigan or Ohio or whatever, but their definition of winter was going from the warm car to the ski slope, playing in the sun while wearing thousand dollar snowboard pants, drinking some hot cocoa back in the lodge and spending most of the rest of the winter in the house playing Nintendo because they were raised by women. Meanwhile, I thrived because while yes, I am from Texas, I'm from the Panhandle where we get blizzards and ice storms that will curl your hair. More importantly, my dad had me running the pressure washer at the mower shop when it was 35 degrees and overcast every goddamn day. Snow? Bitch, please. The Marine Corps gave me Gore-Tex pants, which beat the ass off the Levi's I grew up in (that would actually be Rustlers, the Wal-Mart knock off Wranglers, if you want to be precise). Actual waterproof gloves too? Shieeeet. All I gotta do is pull this heavy ass sled with my snowshoes on and point my rifle the way Big Sarge says? Fuck man, I'll do this every winter. You bet your ass I wasn't shy about reminding those shivering bitch boys where they were from every time they started sniveling out loud.

I also saw one of the funniest things I've ever witnessed, which has nothing to do with the chapter but I'mma tell it anyway. We did have one dude in the platoon who was no shit from Jamaica. Early on, I walked outside the barracks one day to find him wearing every piece of cold weather kit we were issued looking like Ralphie's little brother from *A Christmas Story.* He turns to me and says in a chattering Jamaican accent, "I'm freezing my f-u-u-u-c-k-i-n-g aaaaassssss off, mon!" I almost died.

Anyway, my point is that where you grew up has little to do with it. Now there are some jobs that statistically do make hardcases; cowboys, iron workers, roughnecks, those guys tend to be tough. I grew up around them and in my personal experience it tends to be true because they work outside in all conditions, and it's a job that lends itself to keeping going, injured or not. That is a rarity in our world. While it isn't always true in these cases, it tends to be. If you do any of that for a living, feel free to skip this chapter.

Another point I want to bring up is a commonly held belief among my retired friends. The saying is, "I don't have to practice suffering." It's easy to think that if you've lived the life we lived. However, I have to disagree somewhat. I am nowhere near as hard as I was seven years ago when I retired. I know this because I notice things like rain falling on me when I go to the chicken coop or wishing I had brought a thicker jacket. That's something different than being an Amphibious Commando and putting on the wet swim cammies from last night the first thing this morning so you don't have to launder another set—after you break the ice off of them. Now I am not going to go lay in the mud holding perfectly still and watching my backyard just to see if I still can, but I am going to take my own advice in this chapter and start working on my mental toughness just to sharpen it up. I recommend you do the same. For what is coming, mental toughness trumps almost everything else. If this sparks off, suffering is going to be a common denominator.

To start, if you are pussy or suspect you might be a pussy, the first step is acknowledging that you would like to change that about yourself. Self-awareness is a huge bit of self-improvement and something a great many egos can't handle. If you are ever going to make a change in your life, you have to start out with a desire to do so. Then, incremental improvement. There is some military science to this and decades of experience proving it works. I'm not talking about things like a Special Operations Selection, that is a different animal. An environment like that is built purely to separate the wheat from the chaff and they don't give a fuck about helping you succeed. The first day there may in fact be your worst. I'm talking about something like all the way back at basic training.

This is not a well-known fact but since about the mid '80s, you can just quit boot camp. Seriously. No harm no foul, not even a bad discharge. It's just like you never showed up in the first place except that you are barred from ever coming back. Basic Training does have a vested interest in making everyone that could possibly be a soldier into a soldier, Marine, Airman or whatever. They already spent time and money bringing you to Ft. Benning or MCRD Parris Island and they have a certain number of output that is required. Now what would happen if they just chucked everyone in a frozen duck pond for a couple hours on Day 1 followed by some log PT and an all-night ruck march? By the next morning, they would have about 5% of what they started with. Most people are in no way ready for that coming off the street, but if you build them up they can be.

So you start small. You start by doing something that is a little bit uncomfortable for you. Maybe you take a cold shower once a week. Maybe you skip lunch on Wednesdays. You figure out approximately where the limit is for you and then try to do that plus a little more every time. Mental toughness is like cardiovascular ability. If you build it over time, you will be surprised by how good it can get.

I use cold and hunger as good starting points because both of those will easily make cowards of a man. If you have never been wet and cold for an extended period of time, it sucks. Wet and cold is a common denominator of every US Special Operations Selection that I know of. Be it surf torture at BUD/S, swimming the creeks at Ft. Bragg for SF selection or night time hydrographic surveys at ARS, everyone has figured this out. US Army Ranger school is arguably the hardest course in the DOD in terms of physical punishment and even they have a special regard for Rangers that are stupid enough to go and graduate the winter classes. It wasn't uncommon years ago for them to sew their Ranger tabs on with white thread, an indicator even among their peers.

Hunger is another beast and it is a safe bet to say that most Americans have *never* been anything close to truly hungry. What is the longest you have ever gone without food, not a single calorie? By even the third day, the physical effect is very real and your senses go mad. You can not only smell a cheeseburger from five miles away but your brain will start making up fake smells to boot. The first time you experience hunger, you will realize that in that moment you can think of nothing else but food. At least, without a built in armored core of discipline. At any military training where hunger is a built in challenge, the tempers get short. Stealing food is an instant dismissal and yet it still happens.

How do you counteract these forces? Experience, for one. Now this can easily go overboard, so reign it in. A temporary calorie deficit for a young man is an inconvenience, while for an older man it can be a dangerous crash of blood sugar levels. Same with the cold; learning to deal with the cold isn't something that should cost you toes to frostbite like this is North Korea or something. But you can start taking baby steps, like building in some time each week to be hungry and cold. Isn't this a barrel of fun?

Fatigue is absolutely something else that can make you a coward. Not only the sleep deprivation kind, but the just being run ragged kind. This is a hard thing for non-veterans to believe, but you can be so wasted from a very long gunfight that your body just wants to quit, even if that means dying. I'm talking about taking zero damage from bullets but being absolutely wasted just from running around and shooting back. It sounds crazy but it's true. Eventually all those adrenaline chemicals run out and wear off, it's usually hot for good measure, and you are just so physically tired that you don't want to play anymore, consequences be damned. The only things that will keep you going are the will to live, which usually comes from faith (be it God, the cause, whatever), and a desire to win. Those SOF type selection courses are so hard on you especially because of the latter. They need to make damn sure that your will to win is higher than your wish to quit ever could be. Trust me, I was in a firefight so long once that my abs cramped up from changing angles to shoot out of the truck.I had to switch hands because my finger couldn't pull the trigger anymore. Only an iron will kept me going and I'm glad I had it. If any one of my teammates hadn't had the same, I have zero doubt we would have been overrun and slaughtered.

Fortunately, there is an easy builder for this one. Physical training is great because it trains you to work against exhaustion, cold and pain. Every time you go for a run or walk in the rain and go farther than you thought you could, you put a little "don't quit" in the tank. When you go out to your cold ass garage and lift before bed, even though it's late and you are tired, you get a little more.

This is also one of the reasons I love combat sports and why I preached about their value so much in *Concrete Jungle*. They teach you things you can learn from few other places about having fire in your heart and battling on through fatigue. Even now, I get so worn out rolling with the young assholes with good cardio that sometimes I want to quit and go home, but I don't because I have too much pride. Wrestling with another man who is absolutely kicking your ass will take you to a place of physical exhaustion that is hard to reach otherwise. Finding the will to keep fighting and to not let him have an easy submission so you can breathe for a minute, builds character like nothing else I have experienced. Highly recommended.

You need all that "don't quit, fight on" in the tank that you can get because it is highly probable that one day the chips will really be down and you will need all of it you can muster. It may be you all shot to shit, just trying to hang on, or one of your buddies and you have to keep carrying him fast enough to escape a pursuing enemy. The military is full of stories of dudes doing incredible shit, such as Braxton McCoy's tale of survival and then nearly a decade of rehabilitation just to walk again, or MSG Scott Ford at the Battle of Shok Valley, fighting on for hours with his left arm dangling by threads of muscle and most of his team wounded. Any such tale, I can guarantee you this: whoever is featured was a hard motherfucker to begin with and they had to find new reserves within themselves to make it. Mental strength cannot be overstated as an asset.

For a good resource on fitness available on the interwebs, Drew Baye's High Intensity Training is fantastic. He is on the highly recommended list. Not only does he know what he is doing, he can help you avoid idiotic injuries from incorrect lifting. Drew has spent a lifetime studying what does and doesn't work, as well as the how and why to use certain exercises.

Having a few odds and ends around the house is also a pretty cheap option for training. I frequently use a Suples Bulgarian Bag, which will absolutely smoke your balls off. Add a couple kettlebells and an ab wheel and you are in business.

14   Pinch of This, Dash of That

A common maxim of logistics attributed to Napoleon has never been more true: "Amateurs discuss tactics. Rank amateurs discuss Grand Strategy. The professionals discuss logistics." In many ways, this sums up modern warfare. You might occasionally get around some of it, and money and stuff is no guarantee of a successful outcome, but the ability to move and have "stuff" does matter, without question.

This chapter deliberately comes before guns and ammo because not only is this more important, but it is harder to grasp. Look, it's super easy to have a Rambo fantasy about using a mountain of bullets to blast all the bad guys then sit down for a nice Christmas dinner. Reality says that while fighting implements are important, they are usually not the most important. The two counter balance. On the one hand, you aren't protecting shit without a gun and something to feed it, so your pile of Ramen just became their pile of Ramen without it. On the other hand, if you haven't seen anyone to shoot in four months and your kids are hungry, you may wish you had a little less Russian steel case 7.62x54R and a little bit more Spam.

Going into this, I am also fully ready to admit that I don't have all the answers. Not just because you will have different logistical needs based on your AO, but because even with twenty years of thinking about this, I still don't consider myself an expert. Even eight months ago when the COVID thing was plaid and I locked my family in the house for a month, thirty days showed some weaknesses in my ability to plan ahead. It was nothing Earth shattering that we couldn't overcome, but some lessons were definitely learned on what I could have done better. That is probably true for some of you as well. In that regard, COVID was also something of a gift. We learned not only about our own resources but how easily the nation's logistics train could break down and what items are likely to be gone when a new crisis breaks out. Even as someone that tracked where things came from pretty well, I was surprised by some of the stuff that just ceased to exist.

Let's call this a broad overview with some things you may not have thought about. As you recognize weaknesses in your own plans, I suggest you then seek out experts in that field to supplement your knowledge. I can tell you what you may have missed, but I also turn to the prepping community at large for things that are not in my area of expertise. I also realize that stocking up could be very expensive and some of us have been badly hurt economically this year. This isn't a hard and fast 'buy everything on the list' thing because that is unrealistic for many of you. Most preppers spend years getting their stuff together, and I hope you started early. If you didn't, take the time to think through your personal needs before you go spending what little resources you have.

Food

I'm going to start with what I feel is the biggest logistical need and the one that requires the most explanation. This was easy for the urban book; they don't have that much storage and the best move they can make is to leave. You however, as we postulated earlier, have nowhere left to run. I am suggesting a year's supply of food on hand and two if you can possibly swing it.

Wait a minute, the memes I read all say that "Red Counties make all the food." We have all the cattle and wheat, LOL, we gonna be fine! Yeah, not so much. While that is true right now for the most part, things have a nasty way of changing. War is destructive as hell and it is very easy for our surplus to become collateral damage. Before we even get into that, let's look at the logistics of farming and ranching.

First of all, farming is a lot more complex than ex-mayor Michael Bloomberg would have you think: "You dig a hole, you put a seed in, you put dirt on top, add water, up comes the corn." Yeah, not so much. I have cousins that are at least 6th generation farmers that we can trace back in this country. They may be 200th generation farmers for all we know. The task is not easy. It is true that for a pound of produce on the scale, thanks to mechanization and other technology, it takes less man hours now than it ever has in the past. But that mechanization and tech comes at a price. There is all kinds of crazy shit that goes into the profession outside of seeds made in a lab and the science of planting cycles, like field nets and wi-fi enabled irrigation systems that let one man with a phone do what used to take ten with a pickup truck.

The same goes, in some ways, for ranchers. While it might still be an incredibly hard job, at least on the bigger operations, tracking collars, drones, etc. have made it so that less humans are required per animal. All of this is susceptible to breaking apart during things like a Civil War.

Outside of the tech, you still have issues like fuel, medicine, feed and all the logistical web that keeps a modern farm or ranch productive. But don't cowboys just use horses? Sure, sometimes, but you show me the rancher that doesn't have a flatbed truck for moving hay, or the one out west that doesn't have water troughs filled by a tanker truck. Just a crunch in the supply of diesel big enough and long enough would have a devastating effect on livestock herds. If push comes to shove, that rancher is going to have to pick which cows live and which die. This means the surplus we are accustomed to may be over with.

For farmers, we run into three problems in the same vein, without even exercising all the possible shenanigans. Just the combine used for harvesting is a potential disaster for a year's harvest. Fuel, obviously; without fuel for both the combine and the trucks used to get a harvest from the field, it's game over. It could be much worse. Do you have any idea what a modern combine costs? One of my cousins just priced one, so I do: over a million dollars. $1,000,000-plus for a single machine. That may not even get you the leather seat and heated cup holder option! There are electronics on board that would make a Bentley blush, despite what the coastal politicians might think about us deplorables. So how fragile do you think the spare parts supply chain might be? Are all the parts made in the USA, from raw metal to the circuit board? How about all the critical parts?

Because of the investment needed for such a machine, most farmers don't even own one. A million bucks is a lot of scratch for a machine that you use once or twice a year. Instead, the majority of the crops are cut by harvest crews and it's been that way for decades. All my uncles did this in their youth for extra money. A harvest crew is backed by someone that had the money to buy the required trucks and combines up front. Then the local farmers hire them to harvest for a set price. It works out for the farmer because he doesn't hold the note on a million dollar combine, and it works out for the harvest crew because they cut a hell of a lot more than a single farm.

The harvest cycle is basically determined by latitude. Crops are ready to harvest earlier in the South than in the North, which isn't rocket science to figure out, but because of how it is done time wise, it isn't uncommon for a single harvest crew to cut everything from Texas to Montana and the Dakotas. Wait, what? Yes it is entirely plausible and common for the same crew and machines to cut basically everything there is to cut. So what happens if some Uber-Genius Tactician Blue-tard decides to destroy the combines in Texas? You lose everything North of that. It doesn't even have to be on purpose; if enough of the machinery got caught in a crossfire about something entirely unrelated, it doesn't matter. It wouldn't take that much to lose the ability to harvest the majority of the crops in the heartland.

That can also have a cascading effect over into livestock. Assume we lose half the harvest. It could be worse but we still have a lot. Now what percentage of that was normally allocated to livestock that can be converted to human consumption? This is also an easy way for factional fighting to break out among what should have been allies. These assholes want to feed the corn to their people because the people are hungry and disgruntled. These other assholes want to feed the corn to the cows and let the people be hungry and disgruntled for now, but alive through the winter so we have something to eat next year. This is the stuff of nightmares but it isn't implausible.

So yes, I think you should have a minimum of a year of food on hand. That becomes six months of food if you have to also feed the family next door and four months if you include the one down the street. I have faith in the ability of American ingenuity to fix this but it might not fix it fast.

If you are a farmer, you might go looking for some antique equipment just in case. A lot of it can be found in the flower beds of trendy women that own three acre "ranches." Try to find you an old man that still remembers how to work it. Even if you just use it as a hobby on a little patch of ground, you are gaining valuable experience. I hate to think of us going back to the dark ages of horse drawn plows, but it beats going back to hunting and gathering.

Speaking of hunting, what about wild game? Sure man, it's a supplement. I had ten deer in my backyard this morning, but how long is that going to last? Poaching was a huge problem back in the Great Depression. Factor that in with still being a much more agricultural society then and having about one-third of our present population. Game animals basically only still exist in this country because Fish and Game has a huge budget to keep you from eating the King's elk. If that is no longer in play, 350 million hungry mouths will decimate it. Factor in the waste from dipshits shooting anything that moves, half of which is wounded and dies never being found, and the things that will be killed and butchered by chuckle fucks that think steak comes from the factory in a plastic wrapper. Not good. If you yourself are a hunter, this is also a good year to process your own harvest. Not taking anything away from the pros, and they need to stay in business too, but even if you know how, this is a perishable skill. If things going forward get really bad, you might not want to take that red gold into town to have it ground up.

So yeah, food can get pretty plaid. How are you going to prep for this? The Mormons are an outstanding resource who will help even you Gentiles. Seriously, they have a store with supplies online that is open to everyone, not just church members. The Magic Underwear Team are the original gangsters at this; they play for keeps. The amount of knowledge concerning food storage at your local LDS Temple is mind boggling. Not to mention, in my experience, Mormons make really good allies anyway. They have no qualms at all about killing a heathen but they are also very nice and very knowledgeable.

If you can swing it, a solar system with a battery just big enough to run a deep freezer isn't a huge investment. Even one split between two or three families could make a big difference. A refrigerator consumes a lot more juice but I wouldn't rule it out.

Water

Again, this is region dependent. If you live in a town just east of Las Vegas, you probably want to get some 55 gallon drums at the least and a cistern if you can afford it. I have a duck pond in the backyard and I'm a rifle shot to a creek, so it's not such a big concern.

What is a concern for all of us however is purifying that water. The double edged sword of living among a high concentration of livestock is that while there might be water available, it 100% has giardia and other cryptosporidium in it. You will need to be able to purify it. I use a Berkey water filter for the house, following the fact that it is very popular among missionaries going to the 3rd world. The Berkey is great for purifying relatively large quantities of water. You could get away with one of these per four families if you bought the big one, which drives the cost down a lot. For your backpack, I recommend the $20 LifeStraw or a Katadyn pump.

Fuel

Now this is a doozy. Having lots of fuel (gasoline, kerosene, diesel) for machinery on hand would be great, because outside of places like Borger, Texas and a few other little places in Montana I know of with both raw supply and a refinery, the rest of us are in a pickle. It is very conceivable that the fuel supply gets cut off, either by tactical decision or just in the chaos. Fuel is very hard to move in a place with rockets flying willy-nilly. I personally thought the guys driving the fuel convoys across Iraq were probably the ballsiest sons of bitches in the theater. Imagine taking a mile long convoy of Mad Max tanker trucks full of gasoline across 400 miles of IED strewn desert—they actually did it.

Further complicating the issue, fuel does eventually go bad. Gasoline has a shelf life of about six months, which is a shock if you have never heard that. Fuel stabilizers can in theory extend that to three years but you are still gambling. Diesel previously lasted a year and a half or two years with nothing added, but recent data suggests it now starts changing at the molecular level in as little as 28 days after refining. Neither of which is great if we are talking about a long term solution.

Many farms and ranches have large, above ground baby fuel farms already. These maybe hold 600 gallons or so, which is a lot if you drive a Prius to work, not a lot if you need to fuel tractors, trucks, generators and all the fun stuff. They are not, however, terribly expensive all things considered. A 550 gallon tank will set you back about $1300, then whatever it takes to fill it. If you are friendly with a local rancher, see if he would let your group go in on a spare tank or two. Maybe he gets a price break buying in such large quantities, which would also be a bonus, but having some spare fuel on hand would no doubt be worth the price of the infrastructure to hold it.

If that is off the table, consider what tasks you might need to do right now that you wouldn't want to do with a hand tool. Our old pal "The Safety Doc," Dr. David Perrodin, just laid in nine cords of wood for the winter. I am working on another four myself right now, giving me a two-year supply of heat, because I would rather do it with my chainsaw and truck than with an ax and my kids' wagon.

Cooking and Heating

On that note, if you're in a cold region and you don't have what I call a "mechanical backup" for heating and cooking, get one. In Arizona, you could be happy in a My Little Pony sleeping bag in the house in January. In Idaho and North Dakota, not so much. A mechanical backup is something that works 100% without electricity or fuel that isn't sourced locally. Like, I can get firewood from my back yard in a pinch, I cannot get propane no matter how deep I dig. For heat, this is a fireplace or a wood stove, with the wood stove being much more efficient.

For cooking, yes you can get by with a shopping cart for a grill and a pile of twigs, but it isn't really efficient. I bought a factory-made smoker that allows me to smoke or grill with just wood if needed and I am practicing just that. Better to burn up a pot of rice now while I have McDonalds as a backup than later when I really can't afford to waste food. If we get blown out of our firebase, I'm still gaining knowledge to make that Home Depot shopping cart grill work later.

Medical

A large supply of kerlix and tape goes without saying. You need to be prepared for serious first aid if the ambulance crew is out of fuel and the nearest trauma center is in enemy territory. In addition to an Individual First Aid Kit (IFAK) on your belt or chest rig, you need a bag of goodies. Our friends at SOLATAC are a good resource, as is your local Walgreens, but this goes beyond first aid.

Have you ever had athletes' foot, jock itch or a hemorrhoid? How much fun do you think that would be without some meds to cure it? The same goes for day to day minor issues that we can fix with ease thanks to our local Wal-Mart. Think about what you have needed in the past, what is probable and what was unavailable during the COVID scare. From hand lotion to Tylenol, you need a supply. I recommend the Costco sized generic painkillers and vitamins if you have the extra coins. I also strongly recommend *The Ultimate Survival Medicine Guide* by Joseph and Amy Alton. He is an MD, she is a nurse, and over the last decade they have done all kinds of *crazy* self-testing with off the shelf antibiotics and whatnot sold for animals. This means you can buy them without a prescription. This isn't some lady killing her husband with fish tank cleaner, it's legit. This is rather a must have book.

Anything else? I do also recommend some, uh… *grass seed*. Even if you don't partake of the Devil's Lettuce recreationally, you should by now be able to understand its role in pain management. It's not as good as morphine but morphine is harder to grow. I'm not suggesting you raise a crop right now while the DEA still cares, but the second the revolution starts, you bet your bottom dollar I will have a field of nature's own on tap.

Other

What did we learn was hard to get during the COVID hoax? Get some of that. Anything made overseas, including overseas materials, will be very hard to resupply. I was an early adopter of getting my kids two sizes up in shoes—room to grow—and for me, since I wear a size 14 boot, I also secured a couple of extra sets. Dog food, chicken feed, get anything you can think of that would be very hard to get and nice to have if the trucks shut down.

Since hygiene has a direct effect on your overall health, you'll need cleaning supplies. Extra toothpaste and dental floss; have you ever not had some dental floss and needed it? Imagine a thing stuck in your teeth *forever*. This is cheap and easy. Dental floss is also great for sewing nylon back together (thank you, cheap ass USMC supply system).

The sky is the limit here but resources aren't. Do the best you can with what you have available.

15   Myths Will Get You Killed

I hate to break your heart but I'm going to: the odds are extremely high that you can't shoot for shit. Wait, what? Isn't that part of rural culture? It's in all the songs, it has to be true, right? No it doesn't. Are there exceptions to this rule? Varmint shooters tend to not suck; shooting woodchucks at 1000 yards is a pretty precise game. Anybody high level at trap and skeet has some skills. But those are the anomalies.

Let me authenticate this here via story time. In addition to growing up on that dirt road, I got my first rifle when I was 11 years old. Like many of you, I kept it under my bed. That was my shit and my allowance was frequently bricks of 22LR that I shot the absolute piss out off; Federal Lightning in the blue and gold box. I thought I could bang because I could do things like shoot a golf ball at 100 yards with my iron sights. Don't ask me how many rounds that took because it wasn't something I would have even thought about at the time. Then I went to USMC boot camp, we got to the rifle qualification part and I left the 500 meter line with the Pizza Box of Shame: the USMC Marksman badge. Mother Corps has three levels of qualifying with a rifle, in descending order: Expert, Sharpshooter, and Barely Fucking Passed, err... I mean Marksman. It turned out I actually couldn't shoot for shit either, and it took me a lot of hard hours to turn that weakness into a strength.

"But I've been doing it for twenty years!" Cool story, bro. You can do something wrong for twenty years (or fifty years), especially if there is no consequence to doing it wrong and no idea that it can be done better. "But what about those country boys that showed up and could already shoot their asses off?" You mean, of course, Alvin York and Carlos Hathcock. True, but they're exceptions to the rule. Odds are also good that you are not Alvin York or Carlos Hathcock.

Look, I'm not just pulling this data out of my ass or assuming that because I sucked, everyone must suck. In the subsequent years, I ended up teaching a lot of marksmanship, and Hathcock reborn with natural talent on loan from God has yet to show up. I see terrible shooting all the time: dudes zeroing a deer rifle on a milk jug at 25 yards and bros blasting away at a tin can close enough to kick, missing with a whole magazine. The desert around Boise is rife with good ol' boys making noise and not much else. It is actually painful to watch sometimes.

The point is some half-assed shooting isn't going to be good enough as this progresses. It might be sufficient early on when the other side couldn't hit the broad side of a barn from inside it either, but as Tactical Darwinism chews up and spits out the weak, it is going to be more and more of a handicap. The best thing you can do is get some professional help. Scrape the pennies together and go take a class from someone competent. FieldCraft Survival is all dudes I know from the Army and they are as legit as it gets. A Kevin Owens long range class will change your life. There's a myriad of other retired SOF ninjas that are out there teaching right now.

If that is out of the question, then consider going to a local match and even just watching. 3 Gun, USPSA, whatever, the people will be friendly and will answer questions if you have them. If I were to encourage you to take up a sport or pick a local Rabbi, it would be from PRS. Those are the best rifle shooters in the world right now and anyone playing in the top half of that sport is going to know his shit.

Just like a lot of other things we covered, the first step is knowing you have a weakness. Really, you have nothing to lose. If you show up at a match with your deer rifle and kick everyone's ass, then I was wrong. But take the time to find out before you find out the hard way.

16 Guns, Knives, Sharp Sticks, Tactical Nukes

This chapter is almost a cruel joke as of October of 2020. With bare shelves and elevated prices, you mostly got what you got. However, we may have longer than a few months before this sparks off and supplies may normalize a bit in the meantime. So in deference to *Prairie Fire* standing the test of time, I'm including it anyway. If ammo scarcity causes you to weep, feel free to skip this part until such a time as you can buy a pallet of 9mm for eleven cents per round again.

The section on guns and ammo is last by design. While you do need something, the fallacy is often to overdue this category. You cannot buy a victory. An offset of better equipment or money spent is rarely going to be the deciding factor, if ever. If you could win by just having better guns or spending more money on them, we would have dominated Afghanistan twenty years ago, Vietnam fifty, and Korea eighty. In each of those conflicts, we outspent our enemy by orders of magnitude and had better individual Grunt "stuff" by a *huge* margin—we still failed to win.

I'm going to put out what I see as my ideal but don't think you absolutely have to have what I say is best. I am merely trying to steer you to the best money spent; bang for the buck. At the end of the day, an SKS with a pocket full of stripper clips is absolutely enough.

When I think about things like recommending guns, I put myself in the situation of asking, "Is there any equipment offset that would cause me to choose someone I don't know over one of my old Teammates?" And the answer is absolutely not. Any of my old Teammates would be a battle hardened, highly skilled, fifteen to twenty year fully trained commando. I'd take one of those motherfuckers with a Detective Special and a steak knife, or drunk and mostly naked, for that matter.

I'm using the SKS as a base example precisely because it is such a bullshit gun compared to a modern battle rifle. Designed in 1943 while the Soviets were still up against the ropes by the German offensive, it is an unholy combination of plywood and stamped metal. It has a shit trigger, laughable accuracy and doesn't even feed off a detachable magazine, but (and this is a big but) it is a semi-auto, it shoots a lethal bullet, reloading it via stripper clip is reasonably fast and it is as reliable as the day is long. If the AK-47 is the peasants' rifle, the SKS is the poor peasants' rifle. Still, it is absolutely, 100% enough.

I also want to dispel a couple of myths up front. One myth is that having a pile of guns matters—it doesn't. I hear dumb shit all the time like, "Man, you have a lot of gats. Whoever has the most guns wins, amiright? Nobody better mess with you!" I can only hold one at a time and I'm a lot more concerned about the guy that has one gun; he probably knows how to use it. Also, life is not a video game. There is another fallacy out there that you are going to have all these specialized weapons and pick your load out based on the mission at hand. You have to have a sub gun and a carbine and a sniper rifle and fifteen variants of pistol and a shotgun and we are gonna go to the arms room after the Warning Order to get our shit right for the job! No, that's absolutely not real life. I have been in military units with an arms room that would make *Call of Duty* blush and even with access to all this whiz bang shit, a real war rapidly showed us that most of it was silly at best. Ask any SOF veteran you might meet what gun he carried. 99.9% of the time, the work got done with his M-4, which is essentially an AR-15 with an extra hole for the auto seer that he never once used (this is excluding belt fed machine guns, which neither you nor I have access to anymore).

A big pile of guns, in real combat terms, is money you could have spent better elsewhere. After you equip yourself and any family members big enough to use one, everything else is a collectible Pokemon for all intents and purposes. If I had to leave my house *today* because we are being overrun, I'm taking one rifle and maybe a pistol. If I need to start shedding weight, that pistol is among the first things to go.

There is an absolutely stunning graphic floating around that I wish I could include right here. I can't find the owner of it, so I'll spell it out instead. The top block is a fully decked out 1st tier AR-15 with all the best additions you can make: IR laser, high quality optic, suppressor, aftermarket trigger, etc. This block also includes a set of PVS-14 night vision goggles, a mid-tier but good pistol (P320, Glock, whatever), a belt kit and a helmet. Price tag: $10,000, which many will balk at. The next block contains five shit tier shotguns, a couple of off brand pistols, a couple of cheap rifles and several Chinese knock off red dots and scopes. Price tag: $10,000, which is the block owned by a great many dudes that are into guns! The point is, the top block is a higher initial investment per item but overall is *much* better money spent.

Alrighty, let's get to it. Open up the checkbook, here we go! What to start with? Well, prepare for some more heartbreak if your tactical knowledge comes from pressing the X button to sprint. You don't really need a pistol. In terms of combat, a pistol is about as important as the color of your underwear—maybe less important actually. A pistol has about half the ammo capacity of a rifle, the bullets do one-quarter the damage per round and the lethal range is about one-tenth the distance. Professionals can make some incredible long range hits with a pistol, but we are talking about normal human ability here. A pistol takes about four times the hours and ammo to master compared to a rifle, at least. A pistol is mostly used in real armed conflict as a decoration for officers and to execute political prisoners if you happen to be a Commie. They absolutely do not matter 99.99% of the time.

But aren't all the pictures you see of cool dudes in the GWOT showing them carrying pistols? Most of this conflict has been Close Quarter Battle oriented, meaning we go to their house and kill them inside of it. In such a very limited environment, a pistol is faster to unholster than say, clearing a jam in a rifle or reloading one. All true if we are in a gunfight three feet apart. That narrative changes if our firefight is at 200 meters. In such a case, only a fool would whip out his six shooter instead of seeking cover to reload or fix a jam. As you should be avoiding CQB fights at all costs, a pistol is again nearly useless.

While it is much more important to your urban brethren, you might still choose to get one. For the urban dweller, the fight is likely to start with elevated crime and an environment where he can't just be seen going about armed; he needs a pistol. You, in the build up to the real festivities, may also want a pistol for things like going to town, trips to resupply from a Blue but not yet hostile area, etc. I will also grant that a pistol is easier to carry when doing chores like building a fence or skinning a deer. It may pay in the future to always have something on you and a pistol is okay for that.

If I'm going to recommend anything for an all purpose, does everything well, one and done pistol, it's the new class of what I call hybrid size or 1.5 stack pistols. These guns are small enough to be concealed carry everyday, yet through the magic of engineering they shoot like a larger pistol. Despite their tiny size, they have a capacity on par with the last generation of compact pistols and generally double the capacity of sub-compact or slim frame CCW guns of the last gen. Here, you have two choices, both of which are excellent: the Sig Sauer P365/P365XL or the Springfield Armory Hellcat. I even give the Hellcat a slight edge here in proven durability and I would know: I ran 10,000 rounds through a single gun in a weekend as a test for Springfield Armory, and it ate it without so much as chipping the paint. The Hellcat holds thirteen and the P365 holds twelve, both of which are adequate for a do everything pistol.

Outside of those two, just pick one. Most guns today, even the cheap ones, are durable and reliable. Glocks have a shit trigger but are by far the most popular pistol on Earth with aftermarket accessories galore. M&P are an excellent choice and hard to beat with an Apex trigger drop in. The Sig P320 series is stunning and absolutely killed it on reliability during DOD testing. I recommend the X-Series, either X5 or X-Carry. The X guns have a better trigger and a more ergonomic frame than the regular P320 guns. The Springfield Armory XDM family are underrated guns. They're highly accurate and, with the custom shop trigger job, by far the best trigger of any polymer. Springer Precision can also put in a trigger down to nearly two pounds, which beats all but a custom 1911 trigger. The XDM is also a clear class winner if you want a large frame gun, e.g.: a 45 ACP or 10mm. FNH makes an amazing pistol, in the 509 series. After that, Canix makes a fantastic gun for the money. SAR USA makes a $350 CZ-75 clone that is stunning for the price. Grandpappy's 1911 from the war, it really doesn't matter.

Before you buy, go find a holster first. Personally, I won't buy a gun if Safariland doesn't make an ALS holster for it. Since your pistol matters so little, the point is you can buy even a cheap one and be fine.

Alright, rifle time. This matters a little more but once again we live in the Golden Age of weapons. Even what I call a shit tier AR is probably more accurate than my DOD issue M-4, at least before we got some SOCOM specific upgrades in about 2007. My first choice for a rifle would be an AR-15. This isn't the time for exotics and to be different, it's the time to buy the most effective tool. An AR-15 is an M-4/M-16 minus the third hole in the receiver for the full auto or burst sear. If they have enough budget to choose, every commando unit on Earth carries an M-4 or its direct variant, regardless of what they issue the conscripts in their regular Army. This is still true even of the Israelis for all their bullpup bullshit, as well as the Brits. The AR-15/M-4 is the best weapon available on Earth today, so pick that if you can.

ARs come in a wide variety of qualities and prices. The difference in quality usually is going to come down to accuracy and some other minor details. For instance, a very high-quality gun will have a barrel in it capable of producing accuracy that would shame a blueprinted sniper rifle from even twenty years ago. That is not exaggeration; I have a Daniel Defense gun that will shoot groups nearly four times as tight as what was an acceptable one inch standard for an M40A1 circa 2001. In addition to accuracy, the more expensive gun barrels tend to have treatments or coatings that will extend its service life. A good barrel and a cheap barrel might conceivably shoot the same accuracy on day one, but the good barrel is likely to last two to five times longer than the cheap one. A top tier AR is generally also going to have better quality control. If your reputation is made on durability and quality, you will not let an incorrectly heat-treated bolt out the door. A less expensive gun may have cut corners on checking; you might get lucky and you might not. I have yet to see an LWRC with a factory defect but cheaper guns, yes. A top tier gun is also more likely to come from the factory with a good trigger, not some mil spec bullshit.

All that said, you have to choose based on your own financials and for most purposes, any one of these will suffice. ARs usually just work, no matter the cost. The list below is not all inclusive, it merely gives examples. Quality *is* usually based on price, but do your homework because that is not always the case.

<u>Top Tier</u> – Daniel Defense, LWRC, Barnes Precision Machine, H&K, CMMG 300 series – This class will set you back about $2000 but it needs nothing to be fully functional.

<u>Mid Tier</u> – Ranging from the Springfield Armory Edge & Victor, Sig Tread, Barnes Precision Machine (with cheaper barrel option), to the CMMG 200 series – This class of gun is good enough but not perfect. It may need a barrel to be scary accurate, but will likely still do sub inch well within the battle rifle acceptable standard. It may need an aftermarket trigger as an upgrade, but it is a lot bang for the buck. Prices range from around $900 up to $1600.

<u>Poverty Pony or Low Tier</u> – Everything else – Palmetto State Armory, Smith and Wesson, some local brand. It isn't going to have the coolest features and at the really low price end it might actually be outside of spec (over-bored trigger pin holes, off center barrel threading, cheaper metallurgy in the bolt, etc.). Most of it doesn't matter or has a cheap fix: anti-walk pins to keep the trigger in place, a replacement aftermarket bolt, a barrel upgrade later, etc. These are still going to work and likely to be just fine out of the box. Before you get snobby, remember that the Hero of Kenosha looks like he was carrying a Palmetto State shitbox.

For any AR, my first suggestion is to buy a good trigger. A good trigger is an absolute game changer for both speed and ease of hits. The AR Gold from American Trigger Company is absolutely the standard and worth every penny.

Caliber is a little bit of a shooter's choice. The usual question is actually small frame or large frame, referring to the size difference between a 5.56 AR and a 308 size AR. There's a bit of advantage to each, but it largely it doesn't matter. Is one round more lethal than the other? I have a group of friends I still talk to weekly, all of us prior snipers. Several times the question has come up: if you had to do it all over again, would you take an SPR (5.56) or an SR-25 (308). Across our careers, it was about a 50/50 split on what we chose at the time. I was a 308 guy and distinctly remember the first time I shot someone with 308; they fell over like the fist of God hit them—I was sold—but many of my boys used and swear by long barrel 556. Today, I can't tell you with certainty I would pick 308. I'm also older and weaker, which influences my caliber decision, but respectable veterans I know, and whom I know are legit as fuck, make a valid argument for the smaller round.

308 will penetrate barriers better, no question. It also has the advantage of being dual purpose for right now. With a smaller magazine it can be your hunting rifle too. 308 is plenty for deer and legal in states with a minimum caliber restriction. In a pinch, 556 will do that too. I've seen a black bear killed with steel core 556. 22 Magnum is still the poacher caliber of choice, which 556 will vastly outperform. 308 will reach further than 556, if that is a concern. In the same size of gun (308), 6.5 Creedmoor is also an option, which is an easy one mile cartridge, all day long.

308 comes at the penalty of higher weight for the gun and cost per bullet. 308 ammo weighs close to double that of 5.56 per round, so you can reasonably carry twice as much 5.56 all things being equal. That is a big deal. 308, I will grant, uses 30 caliber bullets, the most common to find in the nation. However, for loaded factory ammo, I guarantee there is twice as much 5.56 produced every year. Also, for right now, 5.56 is compatible with nearly 100% of police force armories and military stockpiles. That might matter later. If you want the 308 or 6.5, that is fine too.

Daniel Defense, Larue and LWRC would once again top my list. The Springfield Armory Victor 308 is the best value on the market if you are short on coins.

Usually next in line is an AK-47. I don't personally care for AKs because the ergonomics suck and they don't play well with modern stuff like holographic sights. You can find solutions, but at the end of the day they just weren't made for it. This is only my opinion though. I will concede that an AK is tough, reliable and pretty inexpensive. I do think very highly of the AK's round, 7.62x39mm, for both lethality and barrier penetration. It lacks the range of a 5.56 round but it is nasty inside 300 or so meters.

I will also say that for the caliber, a new hybrid gun exists that is pretty nuts. The CMMG Mk47 is the best mix I have seen yet of an AR style operating system and trigger that feeds off of AK-47 magazines. It is so good that if mine shows up before these assholes start the revolution, I would have a hard time not choosing it as my first line weapon.

Next up is anything semi auto. The M1A family, particularly the Tanker version, is great if you want 308. The Ruger mini-14 isn't a bad choice, though it does tend to lack in accuracy. There's the aforementioned SKS. Then, anything lever action. A bolt action will work if you just can't find anything else.

A shotgun is not my first choice but they are handy for hunting birds, which may be handy as this goes on. While a shotgun is devastating at close range, it is really lacking past about eighty meters without special ammo like flight control buckshot or deer slugs, and a rifle is still better. If I was buying today and I wanted semi auto, I'd get a Beretta 1301 or Benelli M2/M4. If you insist on a pump action: Mossberg 590. Next question.

Okay, with weapons sorted out, what do you need to go with them? I am basing this list on the idea that you got an AR, as that is what I am most familiar with. Not knowing the weak points of other weapons that well, I would be making up a spare parts list.

First, an optic. You don't have to have one but a red dot is easier to learn from scratch if you have no experience. Even the military has folded on that point. Unfortunately, good ones are quite expensive. The Aimpoint Micro T-2 is the king and absolutely bulletproof in durability. They are about $800, which hurts to think about. Next in line is the Trijicon MRO, which I love. Trijicon is known for toughness and this may very well prove to be as good as the Aimpoint, but it is newer so we don't know yet. It costs around $400 or $460 with a mount included. After that, I have no idea. Cheaper options exist but I haven't personally beat any of them up. Holosun has a good reputation but I don't trust anything that cheap. A good rule of thumb here: if you buy the Trijicon or above, you can get the $60 back up irons. If you buy the $60 red dot, go ahead and spend the money for the $200 LWRC steel flip up irons.

AR-15s can and do break. Even the bad ass ones can be damaged by bad ammo, enough time or things going wrong. I would want one spare bolt per five guns. I'd want one spare buffer tube per ten guns, that being a notorious weak point of the AR. Trigger springs break, so have one spare trigger group per ten guns, or just keep the one you pop out when you replace it with an AR Gold. Maybe one spare barrel per twenty guns, in case you lose one to a squib or are so lucky as to burn one out over time. Really, that is about it.

Get all the ammunition you can lay hands to while still buying the other stuff on your list. I recommended that the urban dweller have 1000 rounds, which is also a good start for you. In all the modern conflicts I can think of, everyone wished they had more ammo. A Balkan Conflict urban survivor of the '90s with the pen name Selco talks about this often (shtfschool.com). It can be overdone; 10,000 rounds is no guarantee of victory, especially if you have used none of it for training. I would feel secure with as little as 500 rounds because I have done this before and I can get a lot done with that. I am also past the new guy learning curve where you tend to blast 300 rounds at nothing as soon as the fight starts (some people will never evolve past that. See videos of amazing marksmanship on display in Syria, Liberia or any other recent 3rd world conflict).

The answer here is balance. Ammo may have fantastic trade value later or you may wish you spent it on canning jars instead. The DOD stash may become available either because the Government is arming militias against seditionist guerrillas or things got so fucked up they abandoned it. No one knows how this plays out. Build up a reasonable stash of a thousand or so and don't worry about it if you only have a single basic load. There are a lot of cards still in play and more ammo isn't guaranteed to help.

17   Lions and Dragons and Bears – Oh My!

Allow me now to take a minute and talk about how bad this can actually get. Keep in mind that if I do have a weakness as an analyst, it is that I overthink the enemy's capabilities. Also, I don't have access to classified information anymore so this is purely speculation mixed with open source data. Even if I did, the regions in question are not my area of expertise. However, I do have eyes and I can see, as well as put 2 plus 2 together and find the answer to be 4. The factor we are missing that could possibly play a huge role in the coming conflict is outside interest. This is something that I think the average person tends to miss when they think about what is happening around the world and our nation at the moment.

You have to realize a couple of things. One, countries don't have friends, they have interests. Sometimes those interests align and we pretend to be allies, sometimes they don't and the dominant party forces the weaker party to act against its own interests. Sometimes that becomes a conflict if the dominant party isn't dominant enough to make it an obviously bad idea.

There hasn't been a conflict in a thousand years that didn't have outside parties involved. It may have been covert, it may have been only economic, but there is no such thing as a one vs one war in terms of nations. France sent advisors and some naval support during our Revolution of 1776. England provided safe harbor to the Confederate Navy during the Civil War. The Czar actually sent the Russian Navy to support the Union during the same, which is widely viewed as a flex that kept France and England from intervening directly. For all the good guys vs bad guys rhetoric we espouse today, we did arm the shit out of the Brits well before we entered WW1 and WW2. The Spanish Civil War of 1936 to 1939 had so many foreigners in it that they sometimes had their own units, not to mention on-loan soldiers from the big European players, including air and armor from the Germans to back the Nationalists.

Not only is someone else's war perhaps in your nation's interest, it is a great place to test new weapons. We have done so with items like TOW missiles, first used in combat by the Israelis against Syrian tanks in 1982 with what I am told was an insanely large audience of US General and Field grade officers present to watch. How else are you going to know if it really works against the latest Soviet armor (which happened to be in use by the Syrians at that moment)?

So shit can get really weird, really quick. How could this play out for us? First, who could even muster the strength to do something? Unfortunately for us, most of our allies are only of any possible help in a narrow region. Israel can barely project power to the West Bank, much less West Virginia. There's not enough Brits to matter in the least. What is Japan going to do, send us a container ship of Playstation 6s? Most of our allies are weak sisters, not to mention they are only our allies because we buy them off with billions in foreign aid. While the loss of those billions might incentivize them to try, other forces could be at work that makes the money not worth it.

If we are honest about dogs big enough to make a move, that leaves only Russia and China. I have already seen credible accusations that Chinese money is involved in the BLM and Antifa organizations, which is not a surprise. China plays a long and complicated game by thinking on a time scale we can't fathom. If the opportunity presented itself four years ago to use some useful idiots for no other reason than to destabilize us, would they take it? Of course. While Russia gets thrown around a lot, particularly at Trump the last four years, this also would be something of interest to them.

Isn't it ironic that the Blue Team would actually be a likely culprit for receiving Russian assistance? Tell me that doesn't also fit with what we know about the Radical Left and Alinsky rules. It is often the case in all areas of life that the man howling loudest about his innocence is the most guilty of the crime. The Left loves to play this game with racism, misogyny, respect for law in general, you get the drift. This idea of using idiotic Americans with made up grievances to wreck our nation is straight from the KGB handbook and damn impressively executed if true. Looking at just the command and control elements, not to mention the logistics of current our current "insurgency-lite," I can tell you that this is not organic. It is a controlled operation by someone.

Why wouldn't China and or Russia back this? What does it cost them, a few million bucks? If that sounds like a lot, to those initiated in espionage it's pocket change. A single bureaucracy in a large nation-state spends that on staples and copy paper in a calendar year. If you can inflict a couple hundred million dollars in damage to your enemy by spending only five or ten, that is a gamble worth taking every time. I also want to clarify that I am not postulating China and Russia are in this together. I'm saying one or both, but not coordinated.

Now let's fast forward to how this Red/Blue thing comes apart. Specifically how doesn't really matter; Kurt Schlichter has an excellent set of novels, his *People's Republic* series, if you don't like my scenario. I'm going with Trump wins re-election, Blue Team can't handle it and California, Oregon and Washington secede. We can easily reverse the next sequence by going to other way: Trump wins on election night, Blue Team "finds" enough mail in votes over the next two months to reverse it and the courts uphold it. Red Team refuses to accept the results and Idaho, Montana and Utah secede. The fucked up, plausible and insane thing that could happen is neither team is the clear victor in the election and the Speaker of the House becomes President on Jan 20th. For now, let's go with Blue Team states secede.

Despite the Lincoln Doctrine, there probably isn't the political will to bring Blue secessionists back into the fold by force. So things just brew for a little bit with perhaps a low grade insurgency by the Red Counties in those states. Eventually, Blue decides the insurgency is being fueled by somewhere still in the borders of the United States and they have to act; Fort Sumter all over again. They try an offensive and get their asses handed to them. Red Team rejoices but still lacks the political will to press the victory. Blue Team slinks home and realizes they are out of their depth. So they turn, at the Government level now, to the only ally they can find. China is a natural fit by both coastal proximity and Blue Team desire to have things like social credit scores, party rule and a general thumbs up to communist ideals. China, seeing a chance to take the United States off the playing field for a while, jumps at the chance. They send over weapons and advisors and suddenly Blue Team doesn't suck so bad anymore.

Wait, can't the US Navy stop that from happening? Sure, if someone has definitive control of the Navy. That's a big if depending on how the divorce happens. Who are they supposed to listen to if two separate jackasses are claiming title to the throne? Aside from that, what are they going to do, blockade the port of Los Angeles? We are talking 4th generation warfare here, not an invasion by the PLA in uniform; RPGs and machine guns hidden in container ships full of Amazon shit, not an armada flying the Chinese flag. Are we just going to start sinking every container ship from China? Not likely, and thanks to Hill Dawg we are largely blind in that region.

If China can't actually invade, largely because that would unite Red Team like nothing else, what is in it for them? China is resource poor and they have basically used up all their natural gifts. While they would love to take ours, they don't have the reach. But merely taking us out of the equation gives them a free hand to run roughshod over all of Southeast Asia. We might be able to fight Russia and China at the same time on our best day but we could never fight among ourselves *and* China alone. They would be in this merely to extended the insurgency as long as possible so that they could consolidate gains in their own sphere of influence.

Now if it looks like Blue Team might actually win, what is a good move for Russia? Russia can see two strategic level truths here. First, they cannot allow a Blue Team win in this scenario, as that would be a resurgent United States put on the throne by China. That would be in many ways a United States beholden to and allied with China. Two, they can make the conflict last longer simply by arming Red Team, which allows them the time and space to dominate Europe. Once again, we're not talking a military invasion of Western Europe because they don't need to. After snatching up any former Soviet states they really wanted, they could cause Europe to bend the knee without firing a shot. Europe would still be made up of allegedly free countries but would be vassal states in all but name. Europe is cucked beyond belief already, even with Uncle Sam propping them up. With us out of the equation, capitulation would be a foregone conclusion. Even if they did want to resist, all of Europe combined has about as much military power as a popcorn fart. So let's say Russia sends arms and advisors to Red Team but always just enough to keep Blue Team from winning. How do they get here without ports? Across Canada, the same way they would have done it if the Cold War went hot; very easy reach.

Now we have a proxy war done absolutely perfectly. Russia and China each have their greatest adversary shredding itself at very little cost to themselves. Billions of dollars in weapons and a few thousand advisors lost is nothing compared to all the oil in the North Sea and unfettered control of Southeast Asia. Not to mention, a free hand to fully exploit the natural resources of Africa for a decade or so. All the while they're eating popcorn and watching the Yankees kill each other with guns they gave them. Once we emerge a decade later, we'd find an entirely different world order.

You wanted worse? How about instead of this being adversarial between China and Russia, it was coordinated at the highest levels. Sharing intelligence and materials would help them extend the conflict even longer. It wouldn't even matter if we

154

figured it out at some point; once the killing starts, it is damn hard to stop.

If this starts the other way with Red State secession, we can assume they would quickly be treated like Rhodesia and cut off from recognition or resupply by the rest of the world. However, it's been standing Russian policy for decades, even reconfirmed publicly by Putin not that long ago, that Russia would back any attempt to overthrow the Government of the United States. I think we could count this as something they would back, which ends up with the same results.

Scary stuff but not unthinkable.

18   Advanced Darkness

"This isn't your average, everyday darkness, this is advanced darkness!"

— *SpongeBob SquarePants*

Let me close out here by saying that I don't wish for a war, far from it. I can speak for all of us that fought a war over there, we absolutely do not want a war over here. I for one really like having a truck pick up my garbage, having air conditioning and not worrying about IEDs on my way to pick up a pizza. I'm also not willing to just roll over and lose our nation without a fight.

The situation is dire. It isn't hopeless but it is pretty far from good. We are losing at the moment, which we should all be capable of readily admitting. The consequences of defeat are unthinkable. They do want you broke, dead, your kids raped and brainwashed and they think it's funny. The tranny story book hour of recent years has convinced me that literal demons walk the Earth and it is entirely possible we are for reals ruled by a global child sacrifice pedo cult. Things that were full up tin foil sombrero just three years ago now seem like quite reasonable conclusions.

Blue Team has positioned itself remarkably well over the last seventy years. They have completed the long march through our institutions. They control the media, tech giants, popular culture and a significant portion of the Deep State, including entire Departments. They are primed and ready to conduct 4th and 5th Generation warfare and will win if we let them.

To simplify the terms, 3rd Generation warfare is combined arms mixed with Fire and Maneuver along with bypassing and collapsing enemy forces rather than simply trying to destroy them head on. 4th Generation warfare is basically the use of irregulars, blurring the lines between politics, with the goal of not outright victory but to disorganize and delegitimize the nation in which it is conducted. 5th Generation warfare is that but with economic pressure, heavy on the propaganda via social media, non-state actors without a clear political goal and very little actual violence. There's not a lot of clearly defined lines between the two; one kind of melds into the other. North Vietnam after the Tet offensive is early 4th Gen, the Russian annexation of Crimea is late 4th Gen and the Color Revolutions of Europe are basically 5th Gen.

If you look at the chess board, you will see that Blue Team has in many ways backed us into a corner if we are playing 4th or 5th Gen. However, there is something the egg heads at the think tanks are missing; easy to do if you make up these terms after grad school instead of after a tour in the sandbox. 4th and 5th Gen warfare might be able to do amazing things in the right set of conditions, but they crumble like a sandcastle in a tsunami if they go up against 3rd Gen warfare conducted by people that just don't give a fuck. We did lose in Vietnam despite destroying the NVA because they were able to hang on long enough for us to quit; 4th Gen for the win. How about that Kurdish uprising against Saddam? Oopsie, it doesn't work every time. Why don't the Uighurs revolt in China? Because China would kill them to a man and not blink. 4th and 5th gen warfare loses its teeth if you decide not to care about public opinion or UN binding resolutions.

That is absolutely what I suggest if they push this over into a conflict. You can start right now in the culture war that precedes it. "If you don't support BLM, you are a racist!" Fuck you. "If you don't support teaching anal sex and gender fluidity to kindergartners, you are bigot!" Fuck you. "If you support Trump, you are a literal Nazi!" Fuck you. "If you don't apologize for being born white, you are an oppressor!" Fuck you. "Oh, you engaged in wrong think, now you have to virtue signal like buying an indulgence from the pope!" Fuck you, make me. You have to start standing up to nonsense—now. Mock and belittle this retarded shit every chance you get. People follow strength and it is a good habit to get into for later. Just not giving a shit what people think is a powerful weapon and it's something this country used to have in spades. France won't allow overflight rights to bomb Libya? Fine we will go around. What's that, we also accidentally hit the French embassy in Tripoli? Maybe the pilots were tired... We went from Big Stick diplomacy to Gay Dick diplomacy in a hundred years—Russia mocking our rainbow flag at the Embassy in Moscow is among the most humiliating things imaginable— but the former is still in us.

Remember this: as long as you draw breath, there is hope (*dum spiro spero*). Things are going to get ugly, real ugly, and not just blood and gore but economic destruction and hunger in a way you can't imagine. Get your mind right now. We will emerge on the other side of this.

For me, between now and that day, I'm taking my own advice. I spent a lot of time putting this together at the detriment to my own preparations. It is time for me to work on the cardio, can some fruit and spend some time at the range. I hope we can all laugh about this in the future, but I'm not planning on it.

Time was of the essence, and not everything would fit in the book. I already have things I wish to add, but we have to get the message out now. Check in with me at off-the-reservation.com for updates as the situation develops. Good luck and good hunting, I will see you on the beach!

Printed in Great Britain
by Amazon

49243311R00099